**Pascale Carrington** was born in 1961 in Newcastle upon Tyne, and has lived and worked in Australia and England. She currently lives in London.

# room to love

women write about love, sex and relationships

## pascale carrington, editor

First published by The Women's Press Ltd, 1996
A member of the Namara Group
34 Great Sutton Street, London EC1V 0DX

British Library Cataloguing-in-Publication Data
A catalogue record for this book is available from the British
Library

ISBN  0  7043  4458  0

Phototypeset in Bembo by Intype London Ltd
Printed and bound in Great Britain by
BPC Paperbacks, Aylesbury, Bucks.

*With thanks to Chris Perry*

# PERMISSIONS

The Women's Press would like to thank the following:

Jane Blue, for permission to print 'Room to Love' which is adapted from an unpublished memoir entitled *My Mother and Amelia Earhart*.

Marion Boyars Publishers Ltd, for permission to reprint an extract from *A Time and a Time* by Rosemary Manning, 1986.

Cleis Press, for permission to reprint 'Interview with Debra' by Carole, from *Sex Work: Writings by Women in the Sex Industry* edited by Frédérique Delacoste and Priscilla Alexander, 1987.

Andre Deutsch, for an extract from *Women, Celibacy and Passion* by Sally Cline, 1993.

Farrar, Straus & Giroux, Inc, and Reed Books, for permission to reprint an excerpt from *Break of Day* by Colette. Copyright © 1961 and renewed © 1989 by Martin Secker and Warburg, Inc.

Lucy Goodison, for permission to reprint 'Really Being in Love Means Wanting to Live in a Different World'.

HarperCollins Publishers, Inc, for permission to reprint 'Formulae of Hoodoo Doctors' from *Mules and Men*. Copyright © 1935 by Zora Neale Hurston. Copyright renewed 1963 by John C. Hurston and Joel Hurston.

Dianne Linden, for permission to reprint 'In the Bleak Midwinter'.

Roberta Morris, for permission to reprint 'A Feminist Ovary Goes Its Own Way'.

Oxford University Press, for permission to reprint an extract from *The Paston Letters* edited by Norman Davis, 1963. Copyright © Oxford University Press, 1963.

Alicia Partnoy, for permission to reprint 'Marriage by Pros and Cons' by Clara Piriz, translated by Regina M. Kreger, from *You Can't Drown the Fire: Latin American Women Writing in Exile*, published in the United States of America by Cleis Press, 1988, and in Great Britain by Virago, 1989.

Katha Pollitt, care of Rogers, Coleridge and White Ltd, in association with Melanie Jackson Agency, for permission to reprint 'Not Just Bad Sex' from *Reasonable Creatures*, first published in the United States of America by Alfred A. Knopf, 1994.

Sal and Anne, for permission to reprint 'Stepping Out'.

Scribner, a Division of Simon and Schuster Inc, and The Harvill Press, for permission to reprint lines from 'Last Letter' taken from *Hope Abandoned* by Nadezhda Mandelstam, first published in Russian under the title *Vtoraga Kniga* by Editions YMCA Press, Paris, 1972; first published in the United States of America by Atheneum Publishers, 1972; and in Great Britain by Collins and Harvill Press, 1974. This edition first published by Collins and Harvill, 1989. Translated from the Russian by Max Hayward © 1973, 1974 by Atheneum Publishers and Collins Harvill.

Seal Press, for permission to reprint 'Lusting for Freedom' by Rebecca Walker from *Listen Up: Voices from the Next Feminist*

*Generation*, edited by Barbara Findlen. Copyright © 1995 by Barbara Findlen.

Spinifex Press, for permission to reprint an extract from *The Lesbian Heresy: A Feminist Perspective on the Lesbian Sexual Revolution* by Sheila Jeffreys, 1993.

Alice Walker, for permission to reprint 'Brothers and Sisters' from *In Search of Our Mothers' Gardens*, 1983.

Weidenfeld and Nicolson and The Robert Lantz Joy Harris Literary Agency, for an extract from *Changing* by Liv Ullmann, 1977.

# CONTENTS

# Introduction

In *Room to Love*, women share their passions and desires, their insights and understandings, about love, sex and relationships. Young women, like Rebecca Walker, express a fierce desire to be passionate and sexually active, but also respected and free – choices that have often been contradictory for women. Others – Jane Blue, Rosemary Manning, Alice Walker, and more – look back on early experiences of love and sex with joy, nostalgia and sometimes pain. Married women, in partnership or separated and by choice or by circumstances imposed from without, search for ways to be with their partners in love and equality, despite forces that militate against this. Lesbians describe the particular joys and dynamics that have characterised their relationships.

Letters from Margery Brews to John Paston III poignantly suggest the painful economic realities that have faced women in marriage; other pieces take a wry look at current relationship situations and concerns; and two women write powerfully of the love between mother and child. Finally, Katha Pollitt, Lucy Goodison and Sheila Jeffreys articulate debates about sexual practices and mores.

Here is love, sex and relationships from women's perspectives, as we seek room to love, as ourselves.

Pascale Carrington

# REBECCA WALKER
*Lusting for Freedom*

I had sex young and, after the initial awkwardness, loved it. For days and nights, I rolled around in a big bed with my first boyfriend, trying out every possible way to feel good body to body. I was able to carry that pleasure and confidence into my everyday life working at the hair salon, raising my hand in English class, hanging out with my best girlfriend, and flirting with boys. I never felt any great loss of innocence, only great rushes of the kind of power that comes with self-knowledge and shared intimacy.

But experiences like mine are all too rare. There are forces that subvert girls' access to freeing and empowering sex – forces like Aids, limited access to health care, and advice on contraception that force thousands of young women to seek out illegal and sometimes fatal abortions. The way we experience, speak about and envision sex and sexuality can either kill us or help us to know and protect ourselves better. The responsibility is enormous. Unfortunately, moral codes and legal demarcations complicate rather than regulate desire. And judgements like 'right' and 'wrong' only build barriers between people and encourage shame within individuals. I personally have learned much more from examining my own life for signs of what was empowering for me and what was not, and from listening to and asking questions of my friends: What did you feel then, what did you learn from that?

When I look back at having sex during my teenage years, I find myself asking: What was it in my own life that created the impulse and the safety; the wanting that led me and the knowing that kept me from harm?

If you are a girl, sex marks you, and I was marked young. I am ashamed to tell people how young I was, but I am too proud to lie. Eleven. I was eleven, and my mother was away working. One autumn night Kevin, a boy I had met in the neighbourhood, called and said he had a sore throat. I told him I would make him some tea if he wanted to come over. He said he was on his way. I had told him that I was sixteen, so I ran around for a few minutes, panicking about what to wear. I settled on a satin leopard-print camisole from my mother's bureau and hid it beneath a big red terry-cloth robe.

I have a few vivid memories of that night: I remember being cold and my teeth chattering. I remember his black Nike high tops and red-and-grey football jersey, and the smell of him, male and musky, as he passed me coming through the front door. I remember sitting on our green sofa and telling him rather indignantly that I was not a virgin. I remember faking a fear that I might get pregnant (I didn't have my period yet). I remember his dry penis, both of us looking elsewhere as he pushed it inside of me. I remember that I wanted him to stay with me through the night, but that instead he had to rush home to make a curfew imposed upon him by his football coach.

Shocking, right? Not really. Sex begins much earlier than most people think, and it is far more extensive. It is more than the act of intercourse, much more than penis and vagina. Sex can look like love if you don't know what love looks like. It gives you someone to hold on to when you can't feel yourself. It is heat on your body when the coldness is inside of you. It is trying out trusting and being trusted. Sex can also be power because knowledge is power, and because yeah, as a girl, you can make it do different things: I can give it to you, and I can take it away. This sex is me, you can say. It is mine, take it. Take me. Please keep me.

By the time I was eighteen I was fluent in the language of sex and found myself in restaurants with men twice my age, drinking red wine and artfully playing Woman. By then I had learned about the limitations of male tenderness, men's expectations about black female desire, the taboo of loving other women, the violence of rape. And, like women all over the world, I had mastered the art of transforming myself into what I thought each man would fall in love with. Not at all in control of each affair, but very much in control of the mask I put on for each man, I tried on a dozen personas, played out a dozen roles, decided not to be a dozen people. When Bryan said I was too black, I straightened my hair. When Ray said I was too young, I added four years. For Miles I was a young virgin, nervous and giggly. For Jacob I was a self-assured student of modern art. For Robbie I was a club girl. I was Kevin's steady.

When I think of what determined my chameleon-like identity then, I think of the movie *Grease*, with the dolled-up Olivia Newton-John getting the guy and popularity too after she put on pumps and a push-up bra and became 'sexy'. I also think about my best girlfriend in the fourth grade who stopped speaking to me and 'stole' my boyfriend over Christmas break. It was a tricky world of alliances in those younger years. You could never be sure of who was going to like you and why, and so I tried my best to control what parts I could. That explains my attempts to be cool and sexy, my pretending to know everything, my smoking cigarettes, and of course, my doing it with boys. I did what I thought had to be done.

But there were also other elements, other factors. Like curiosity, desire and my body. These are the urges that account for the wet, tonguey ten-minute kiss outside the laundry room that I remembered with a quivering belly for weeks afterwards. Ditto for my desire to bury my face in my boyfriend's armpits in order to learn his smell well enough to recognise it anywhere. This very same desire to know also made me reach down and feel a penis for the first time, checking almost methodically for shape, sensitivity and any strange aberrations on the skin. My quest was not simply a search for popularity, but a definite assertion of my own nascent erotic power. This strange force, not always pleasurable but always mine, nudged me towards physical exploration and self-definition, risk taking and intimacy building, twisting each element into an inextricable whole.

Because my mother was often away, leaving me with a safe and private space to bring my boyfriends, and because my common sense and experience of non-abusive love led me to decent men, my relationships consisted of relatively safe explorations of sex that were, at the time, fulfilling physically and emotionally. I also began to play with different kinds of strength. While I learned about my partners' bodies, I learned that I had the power to make them need me. While I learned how much of myself to reveal, I learned how to draw them out. While I learned that they were not 'right' for me, I learned that I was more than what they saw.

Did I know then that I was learning to negotiate the world around me and answering important questions about the woman I would become? Probably not, but looking back, it seems obvious: I peeled back endless layers of contorted faces, checking out fully the possibilities of the roles I took on. I left them again and again when I felt I could not bring all of myself to the script. I couldn't just be the football player's cheerleader girlfriend, or the club girlfriend of a bartender. I wasn't happy faking orgasm (self-deceit for male ego) or worrying about getting pregnant (unprotected ignorance) or having urinary tract infections (victim of pleasure) or sneaking around (living in fear). Instinctively I knew I wanted more pleasure and more freedom, and I intuitively knew I deserved and could get both.

When I think back, it is that impulse I am most proud of. The impulse that told me that I deserve to live free of shame, that my body is not my enemy and that pleasure is my friend and my right. Without this core, not even fully gelled in my teenage mind but powerful none the less, how else would I have learned to follow and cultivate my own desire? How else would I have learned to listen to and develop the language of my own body? How else would I have learned to initiate, sustain and develop healthy intimacy, that most valuable of human essences? I am proud that I did not stay in relationships when I couldn't grow. I moved on when the rest of me would emerge physically or intellectually and say, Enough! There isn't enough room in this outfit for all of us.

It is important to consider what happens when this kind of self-exploration is blocked by cultural taboo, government control or religious mandate. What happens when we are not allowed to know our own bodies, when we cannot safely respond to and explore our own desire? As evinced by the worldwide rape epidemic, the incredible number of teenage pregnancies, and the ever-increasing number of sexually transmitted diseases, sex can be an instrument of torture, the usher of unwanted responsibility or the carrier of fatal illness.

It is obvious that the suppression of sexual agency and exploration, from within or from without, is often used as a method of social control and domination. Witness wide-spread genital mutilation and the homophobia that dicta-torially mandates heterosexuality; imagine the stolen power of the millions affected by just these two global murderers of self-authorisation and determination. Without being able to respond to and honour the desires of our bodies and our selves, we become cut off from our instincts for pleasure, dissatisfied living under rules and thoughts that are not our own. When we deny ourselves safe and shameless exploration and access to reliable information, we damage our ability to even know what sexual pleasure feels or looks like.

Sex in silence and filled with shame is sex where our agency is denied. This is sex where we, young women, are powerless and at the mercy of our own desire. For giving our bodies what they want and crave, for exploring ourselves and others, we are punished like Eve reaching for more knowl-edge. We are called sluts and whores. We are considered impure or psychotic. Information about birth control is kept from us. Laws denying our right to control our bodies are enacted. We learn much of what we know from television, which debases sex by humiliating women.

We must decide that this is no longer acceptable, for sex is one of the places where we do our learning solo. Pried away from our parents and other authority figures, we look for answers about ourselves and how the world relates to us. We search for proper boundaries and create our very own slip-pery moral code. We can begin to take control of this process and show responsibility only if we are encouraged to own our right to have a safe and self-created sexuality. The question is not whether young women are going to have sex, for this is far beyond any parental or societal control. The question is rather, what do young women need to make sex a dynamic, affirming, safe and pleasurable part of our lives? How do we build the bridge between sex and sexuality, between the isolated act and the powerful element that, when honed, can be an important tool for self-actualisation?

Fortunately, there is no magic recipe for a healthy sexuality; each person comes into her or his own sexual power differently and at her or his own pace. There are, however, some basic requirements for sexual awareness and safe sexual practice. To begin with, young women need a safe space in which to explore our own bodies. A woman needs to be able to feel the soft smoothness of her belly, the exquisite softness of her inner thigh, the full roundness of her breasts. We need to learn that bodily pleasure belongs to us; it is our birthright.

Sex could also stand to be liberated from pussy and dick and fucking, as well as from marriage and procreation. It can be more: more sensual, more spiritual, more about communication and healing. Women and men both must learn to explore sexuality by making love in ways that are different from what we see on television and in the movies. If sex is about communicating, let us think about what we want to say and how we will say it. We need more words, images, ideas.

Finally, young women are more than inexperienced minors, more than property of the state or of legal guardians. We are growing, thinking, inquisitive, self-possessed beings who need information about sex and access to birth control and abortion. We deserve to have our self-esteem nurtured and our personal agency encouraged. We need 'protection' only from poverty and violence.

And even beyond all of the many things that will have to change in the outside world to help people in general and young women in particular grow more in touch with their sexual power, we also need to have the courage to look closely and lovingly at our sexual history and practice. Where is the meaning? What dynamics have we created or participated in? Why did we do that? How did we feel? How much of the way we think about ourselves is based in someone else's perception or label of our sexual experiences?

It has meant a lot to me to affirm and acknowledge my experiences and to integrate them into an empowering understanding of where I have been and where I am going. Hiding in shame or running fast to keep from looking is a waste of what is most precious about life: its infinite ability to expand and give us more knowledge, more insight and more complexity.

From *Listen Up: Voices From the Next Feminist Generation*, edited by Barbara Findlen, published by Seal Press.

# JANE BLUE
## *Room to Love*

An uncle, my grandmother's last child at home, occupies the sun porch suspended over the back garden. I do not remember his presence. My sister tells me he gave us our breakfast at the painted table in the kitchen, took us to the bathroom in the middle of the night. Daddy has gone off into the silence, and we have moved with Mother into Nana's house.

When my uncle marries, I inherit the room he has vacated, big paned windows facing both south and west, a little garden of nasturtiums and geraniums below, a view of rooftops all the way to the bay. An odd, narrow room with canvas on the floor, it becomes my nest, my haven.

I am four or five, and my life is changed forever because I have this room. My uncle's army cot becomes my bed; across from it there is a student desk and a dresser which Mother paints pink. They are crowded into a little nook by the tiny closet which juts into the room, added on sometime behind the closet in my sister's room. The room is not rectangular, but fits together in pieces like a puzzle. A low bookcase sits under the big windows at the foot of my bed. Mother has papered the walls with big flowers, painted the wood and the canvas of the floor green.

A mirror hangs above the dresser, hidden away behind the closet on a wall that is grooved, some odd and ancient panelling. I see different faces, different selves, when I look in the mirror, trying to decide who I am. This room is where I will live for the next seventeen years, but I always refer to it as my room in Nana's house.

I learn to love myself in solitude.

Nana never catches me, lying on my thin cot, exploring the places in my own body that give me a feeling of love. But when I prepare for confession with the help of a little black book, I decide that this is one of the sins of impurity: *impure thoughts or actions.*

'Alone or with others,' the priest asks in his muffled, face-less voice.

'Alone,' I answer. I do not know which is worse, but I suspect that it is my own sin, the sin of loving myself, alone.

Nana does discover my search for love once, obliquely, not head on. But nothing was ever met head on.

My cousin, who is a year older than I, has come to our house to play, although no one really plays in Nana's house. His mother, my grandmother's oldest daughter, must have dropped him off, for she is not here. She would not leave us together for a moment, as she is the family guardian of morals.

Nana's rule has always been that if we have friends over, we must play in our rooms. We do not have friends, though, because Nana screens them carefully, and no one passes. Cousins are tolerated, as long as we go to my room. We are a girl and a boy, perhaps ten and eleven. My cousin has no sisters; I have no brothers. We are curious.

We decide to practice kissing. In high school, this cousin will have a reputation among the girls as a 'good kisser', so I guess the practice was worthwhile.

What a nice feeling it is as we stand on the green, resilient canvas floor of my room; we are relaxed and warm, and find ourselves lying full length on my little bed, our bodies about the same size, pressed against each other's. I take off my glasses. We grow very, very quiet.

Nana's voice rises, disembodied, disorienting, from down-stairs. She has been working in her study and is glad for the silence, but she looks up from her papers and realises perhaps the extent of it, the vastness that rings into the quiet, loud as a gong.

'What are you two doing up there?'

We get up suddenly. I go to the mirror to straighten my hair.

'Nothing,' I call downstairs in a shaky voice.

After this, I continue to try on selves in front of the mirror, but I do not touch myself, wake myself to myself; I am afraid to leave a mark like the one already on my soul, as they say in the catechism Nana makes sure I attend.

I wrap a white towel around my face to mimic the garb of a nun. I carve the initials of a boy into the grooved panelling. When I look in the mirror, a face stares back, grown and beautiful. I don't know who it belongs to.

I write poetry at my little desk, rushing to get the words down into a composition book with a sewn binding before the feeling passes, an ecstasy as I contemplate the view from my window on a balmy summer night, the full moon illuminating everything like liquid silver spread out on the world, or a silver curtain laid out to dry all the way to the bay.

I cannot describe how I feel any other way:

*The moon shines on bushes and trees, it shines all around, it shines on the sea.*

I remember these words all my life, and the magic of my solitary room comes back to me, and the magic of learning to love.

From *I Am Becoming the Woman I've Wanted*, edited by Sandra Haldeman Martz, published by Papier-Mache Press.

# ROSEMARY MANNING

## From *A Time and a Time*

Very late at night. The meadow at the back of the house is washed empty in the light of the moon, scoured like a shallow bowl. I avoid the paths. Walking on the damp grass under the silver quince trees, and then through the back gate into the road. It's a small town. It takes me only twenty minutes to cross it to the house where she lives, in a room in Mrs Houghton's mock-Tudor villa. The widow Houghton, with sharp eyes and sensitive ears. But I have a duplicate key and have learned to turn a lock without a sound, to tread on the inner side of the stairs, against the wall.

Before I go in, I wait for a few minutes to subdue my heart. I've been walking rapidly. Also I am, for the first time in my life, subject to a strong physical desire that makes my blood throb like drumbeats. I wait, not at the door where someone might see me, but behind the hedge at the side of the house. The air comes cold into my lungs, cold and laden with a heady tang of laurel.

The nights shortened into summer. She slept out in the garden sometimes, and I would step softly in my bare feet under the stars to find her. When they lost their brilliance, I knew it was time to go. On my way home I walk slowly, in step with the dawn, my hair wet with dew.

There's a workman on his bike, riding to some legitimate task. A railwayman, perhaps, or a farm worker. Grey trousers clamped into bicycle clips and a bag at his saddlebar with his sandwiches and tea-flask. He grins in a friendly fashion. She's a collaborator, he thinks, a fellow-traveller up before sunrise.

'Lovely morning!' he calls. 'Lovely morning!'

I'm educated, curse it, my head full of poetry. I pull out a quotation, but for my private ear, not for him: 'The air is all in spice.'

But we do share something: the privileged excitement of being abroad at half-past five on a summer morning, when others are asleep. His cockcrow smile is as good as a line of poetry, any day.

The affair ended disastrously. She left a batch of my letters at her home, in a suitcase, where they were found and read by her parents. Her father, a high official in the church, wrote me a letter threatening me with exposure and legal proceedings. However, he was ignorant of the fact that lesbians cannot be prosecuted. He consulted a lawyer, found out his mistake, and penned another long and blistering letter, admitting his disappointment in the feeble state of the law, but assuring me that he would expose 'my filthy practices' to my employer. He did not, however, carry out his threat. Perhaps he was unwilling to involve his daughter's name. Perhaps he felt that the role of moral blackmailer was inconsistent with his cloth. His daughter was after all in her twenties, and could have defied him. He wrote only once more, to say that the matter was at an end. The whole episode was frightening and humiliating. For a time, while the letters came and had to be read, it also seemed sordid. I was forced to see the affair through an outsider's eyes. Afterwards, when I recalled it, it became our own property again, and we could each evaluate it.

Easter. I am walking along a beach in the early sunshine of the Sunday morning. The sea is very calm, lying supine in the moment of pause between tide and tide, resting thinly over the sands like a wafer on the tongue. And every tamarisk and every clump of sea holly sends a long shadow over the golden sand. Suddenly all my unhappiness drops away from me. I feel overwhelmingly conscious of another's hand clasping my own, the hand of this girl from whom I have only a few days before parted finally. And I am filled not merely with the illusion of her presence beside me but with a benison that pervades my whole being. Perhaps the hand that held mine in its phantasmal grasp that Easter morning was the hand of the life force, that same power that laid the early sun on my skin with its faint but welcome warmth, and drew my eyes to the far out tide that must turn, and the long shadows that must shorten to noon. The power of rocks and stones and trees.

I only saw this woman once again, many years later when she was married and a mother. In the brief moment we were left alone, she suddenly put her arms round me and said: 'I shall never cease to be glad that I knew you and that we loved.' The nightmare that had preceded our parting was washed away finally by this single, touching statement. It was the most graceful ending I have ever known to any affair, though the affair itself was one of the least creditable in my life.

From *A Time and a Time*, published by Marion Boyars.

# ALICE WALKER
## Brothers and Sisters

We lived on a farm in the South in the fifties, and my brothers, the four of them I knew (the fifth had left home when I was three years old), were allowed to watch animals being mated. This was not unusual; nor was it considered unusual that my older sister and I were frowned upon if we even asked, innocently, what was going on. One of my brothers explained the mating one day, using words my father had given him: 'The bull is getting a little something on his stick,' he said. And he laughed. 'What stick?' I wanted to know. 'Where did he get it? How did he pick it up? Where did he put it?' All my brothers laughed.

I believe my mother's theory about raising a large family of five boys and three girls was that the father should teach the boys and the mother teach the girls the facts, as one says, of life. So my father went around talking about bulls getting something on their sticks and she went around saying girls did not need to know about such things. They were 'womanish' (a very bad way to be in those days) if they asked.

The thing was, watching the matings filled my brothers with an aimless sort of lust, as dangerous as it was unintentional. They knew enough to know that cows, months after mating, produced calves, but they were not bright enough to make the same connection between women and their offspring.

Sometimes, when I think of my childhood, it seems to me a particularly hard one. But in reality, everything awful that happened to me didn't seem to happen to *me* at all, but to my older sister. Through some incredible power to negate my presence around people I did not like, which produced invisibility (as well as an ability to appear mentally vacant when I was nothing of the kind), I was spared the humiliation she was subjected to, though at the same time, I felt every bit of it. It was as if she suffered for my benefit, and I vowed early in my life that none of the things that made existence so miserable for her would happen to me.

The fact that she was not allowed at official matings did not mean she never saw any. While my brothers followed my father to the mating pens on the other side of the road near the barn, she stationed herself near the pigpen, or followed our many dogs until they were in a mating mood, or, failing to witness something there, she watched the chickens. On a farm it is impossible *not* to be conscious of sex, to wonder about it, to dream . . . but to whom was she to speak of her feelings? Not to my father, who thought all young women perverse. Not to my mother, who pretended all her children grew out of stumps she magically found in the forest. Not to me, who never found anything wrong with this lie.

When my sister menstruated she wore a thick packet of clean rags between her legs. It stuck out in front like a penis. The boys laughed at her as she served them at the table. Not knowing any better, and because our parents did not dream of actually *discussing* what was going on, she would giggle nervously at herself. I hated her for giggling, and it was at those times I would think of her as dim-witted. She never complained, but she began to have strange fainting fits whenever she had her period. Her head felt as if it were splitting, she said, and everything she ate came up again. And her cramps were so severe she could not stand. She was forced to spend several days of each month in bed.

My father expected all of his sons to have sex with women. 'Like bulls,' he said, 'a man *needs* to get a little something on his stick.' And so, on Saturday nights, into town they went, chasing the girls. My sister was rarely allowed into town alone, and if the dress she wore fit too snugly at the waist, or if her cleavage dipped too far below her collarbone, she was made to stay home.

'But why can't I go too,' she would cry, her face screwed up with the effort not to wail.

'They're boys, your brothers, *that's* why they can go.'

Naturally, when she got the chance, she responded eagerly to boys. But when this was discovered she was whipped and locked up in her room.

I would go in to visit her.

'Straight Pine,'* she would say, 'you don't know what it *feels* like to want to be loved by a man.'

'And if this is what you get for feeling like it I never will,' I said, with – I hoped – the right combination of sympathy and disgust.

'Men smell so good,' she would whisper ecstatically. 'And when they look into your eyes, you just melt.'

Since they were so hard to catch, naturally she thought almost any of them terrific.

'Oh, that Alfred!' she would moon over some mediocre, square-headed boy, 'he's so *sweet!*' And she would take his ugly picture out of her bosom and kiss it.

My father was always warning her not to come home if she ever found herself pregnant. My mother constantly reminded her that abortion was a sin. Later, although she never became pregnant, her period would not come for months at a time. The painful symptoms, however, never varied or ceased. She fell for the first man who loved her enough to beat her for looking at someone else, and when I was still in high school, she married him.

My fifth brother, the one I never knew, was said to be different from the rest. He had not liked matings. He would not watch them. He thought the cows should be given a choice. My father had disliked him because he was soft. My mother took up for him. 'Jason is just tender-hearted,' she would say in a way that made me know he was her favourite; 'he takes after me.' It was true that my mother cried about almost anything.

Who was this oldest brother? I wondered.

'Well,' said my mother, 'he was someone who always loved you. Of course he was a great big boy when you were born

* A pseudonym.

and out working on his own. He worked on a road gang building roads. Every morning before he left he would come in the room where you were and pick you up and give you the biggest kisses. He used to look at you and just smile. It's a pity you don't remember him.'

I agreed.

At my father's funeral I finally 'met' my oldest brother. He is tall and black with thick grey hair above a young-looking face. I watched my sister cry over my father until she blacked out from grief. I saw my brothers sobbing, reminding each other of what a great father he had been. My oldest brother and I did not shed a tear between us. When I left my father's grave he came up and introduced himself. 'You don't ever have to walk alone,' he said, and put his arms around me.

One out of five ain't *too* bad, I thought, snuggling up.

But I didn't discover until recently his true uniqueness: He is the only one of my brothers who assumes responsibility for all his children. The other four all fathered children during those Saturday-night chases of twenty years ago. Children – my nieces and nephews whom I will probably never know – they neither acknowledge as their own, provide for, or even see.

It was not until I became a student of women's liberation ideology that I could understand and forgive my father. I needed an ideology that would define his behaviour in context. The black movement had given me an ideology that helped explain his colourism (he *did* fall in love with my mother partly because she was so light; he never denied it). Feminism helped explain his sexism. I was relieved to know his sexist behaviour was not something uniquely his own, but, rather, an imitation of the behaviour of the society around us.

All partisan movements add to the fullness of our understanding of society as a whole. They never detract; or, in any case, one must not allow them to do so. Experience adds to experience. 'The more things the better,' as O'Connor and Welty both have said, speaking, one of marriage, the other of Catholicism.

I desperately needed my father and brothers to give me male models I could respect, because white men (for example; being particularly handy in this sort of comparison) – whether in films or in person – offered man as dominator, as killer, and always as hypocrite.

My father failed because he copied the hypocrisy. And my brothers – except for one – never understood they must represent half the world to me, as I must represent the other half to them.*

---

* Since this essay was written, my brothers have offered their name, acknowledgement, and some support to all their children.

---

From *In Search of Our Mothers' Gardens: Womanist Prose*, published by The Women's Press.

# KATHA POLLITT
## *Not Just Bad Sex*

'Stick to straight liquor,' my father advised me when I left for college, in the fall of 1967. 'That way, you'll always know how drunk you are.' I thought he was telling me that real grown-ups didn't drink brandy Alexanders, but, of course, what he was talking about was sex. College boys could get totally plastered and the worst that would happen to them would be hangovers and missed morning classes. But if I didn't carefully monitor my alcohol intake one of those boys might, as they used to say, take advantage of me. Or, as they say now, date-rape me.

Veiled parental warnings like the one my father gave me – don't go alone to a boy's room, always carry 'mad money' on a date, just in case – have gone the way of single-sex dorms, parietal hours, female-only curfews and the three-feet-on-the-floor rule, swept away like so much Victorian bric-à–brac by the sexual revolution, the student movement and the women's movement. The kids won; the duennas and fussbudgets lost. Or did they? In *The Morning After: Sex, Fear, and Feminism on Campus* Katie Roiphe, a twenty-five-year-old Harvard alumna and graduate student of English at Princeton, argues that women's sexual freedom is being curtailed by a new set of hand-wringing fuddy-duddies: feminists. Anti-rape activists, she contends, have manipulated statistics to frighten college women with a non-existent 'epidemic' of rape, date rape and sexual harassment, and have encouraged them to view 'everyday experience' – sexist jokes, professorial leers, men's straying hands and other body parts – as intolerable insults and assaults. 'Stranger rape' (the intruder with a knife) is rare; true date rape (the frat boy with a fist) is even rarer. As Roiphe sees it, most students who say they have been date-raped are reinterpreting in the cold grey light of dawn the 'bad sex' they were too passive to refuse and too enamoured of victim-hood to acknowledge as their own responsibility. Camille Paglia, move over.

These explosive charges have already made Roiphe a celebrity. The *Times Magazine* ran an excerpt from her book as a cover story: 'Rape Hype Betrays Feminism'. Four women's glossies ran respectful prepublication interviews; in *Mirabella* she was giddily questioned by her own mother, the writer Anne Roiphe. Clearly, Katie Roiphe's message is one that many people want to hear: Sexual violence is anomalous, not endemic to American society, and appearances to the contrary can be explained away as a kind of mass hysteria, fomented by man-hating fanatics.

How well does Roiphe support her case? *The Morning After* offers itself as personal testimony, with Roiphe – to use her own analogy – as a spunky, commonsensical Alice at the mad women's-studies-and-deconstructionism tea party familiar from the pages of Paglia and Dinesh D'Souza. As such, it's hard to challenge. Maybe Roiphe's classmates really are as she portrays them – waif-like anorexics, male-feminist wimps. Maybe Roiphe was, as she claims, 'date-raped' many times and none the worse for it. The general tone of her observations is unpleasantly smug, but in her depiction of a tiny subculture on a few Ivy League campuses, she may well be on to something. The trouble is that *The Morning After*, although Roiphe denies this, goes beyond her own privileged experience to make general claims about rape and feminism on American campuses; it is also, although she denies this too, a 'political polemic'. In both respects, it is a careless and irresponsible performance, poorly argued and full of misrepresentations, slapdash research and gossip. She may be, as she implies, the rare grad student who has actually read *Clarissa*, but when it comes to rape and harassment she has not done her homework.

Have radical feminists inundated the nation's campuses with absurd and unfounded charges against men? Roiphe cites a few well-publicised incidents: at Princeton, for example, a student told a Take Back the Night rally that she had been date-raped by a young man she eventually admitted she had never met. But Roiphe's claim that such dubious accusations represent a new norm rests on hearsay and a few quotations from the wilder shores of feminist theory. 'Recently,' she writes, 'at the University of Michigan, a female teaching assistant almost brought a male student up on charges of sexual harassment,' because of some mildly sexist humour in a paper. When is 'recently'? In what department of the vast University of Michigan did this incident occur. How does Roiphe know about it – after all, it only 'almost' happened – and know that she got it right? Roiphe ridicules classmates for crediting and magnifying every rumour of petty sexism, but she does the same: hysterical accusations are always being made at 'a prominent university.' Don't they teach the students at Harvard and Princeton anything about research anymore?

Where I was able to follow up on Roiphe's sources, I found some fairly misleading use of data. Roiphe accuses the legal scholar Susan Estrich of slipping 'her ideas about the nature of sexual encounters into her legal analysis' in *Real Rape*, her study of acquaintance rape and the law – one such idea supposedly being that women are so powerless that even 'yes' does not necessarily constitute consent to sex. In fact, in the cited passage Estrich explicitly lays that view aside to pursue her own subject, which is the legal system's victimis-ation of women who say *no*. Nowhere does Roiphe acknow-ledge that – whatever may happen in the uncritical, emotional atmosphere of a Take Back the Night rally or a support group meeting for rape survivors (a term she mocks) – in the real world women who have been raped face enor-mous obstacles in obtaining justice in the courts or sympathy from their friends and families. Nor does she seem to realise that it is the humiliation and stigmatisation and disbelief reported by many rape victims, and documented in many studies, that have helped to produce the campus climate of fear and credulity she deplores. Indeed, the only time Roiphe discusses an actual court case it is to argue that the law veers too far to the victim's side:

> In 1992 New Jersey's Supreme Court upheld its far-reaching rape laws. Ruling against a teenager charged with raping his date, the court concluded that signs of force or the threat of force is [*sic*] not necessary to prove the crime of rape – no force, that is, beyond that required for the physical act of penetration. Both the plaintiff and the defendant admitted that they were sexually involved, but the two sides differed on whether what happened that night was rape. It's hard to define anything that happens in that strange, libidinous province of adolescence, but this court upheld the judgment that the girl was raped. If the defendant had been an adult he could have gone to jail for up to ten years. Susan Herman, deputy public defender in the case, remarked, 'You not only have to bring a condom on a date, you have to bring a consent form as well.'

Roiphe should know better than to rely on a short item in *The Trenton Times* for an accurate account of a complicated court case, and she misrepresents even the sketchy information the article contains: The girl was not the boy's 'date', and they did not both 'admit' they were 'sexually involved'. The two, indeed, disagreed about the central facts of the case. The article does mention something Roiphe chose to omit: the girl was fifteen years old. The Supreme Court opinion further distinguishes this case from Roiphe's general portrait of date-rape cases: the hypersensitive female charging an innocently blundering male with a terrible crime for doing what came naturally and doing it without a peep from her. The offender, it turns out, was dating another girl living in the house where the rape took place, and not the victim, who, far from passively enduring his assault, did what Roiphe implies she did not: she slapped him, demanded that he withdraw, and, in the morning, told her mother, whereupon they went immediately to the police. It is absurd to use this fifteen-year-old victim – who had surely never heard of

Catharine MacKinnon or Take Back the Night — as an example of campus feminism gone mad. And it is equally absurd to suggest that the highly regarded New Jersey Supreme Court, which consists of one woman and six middle-aged men, issued a unanimous decision in the victim's favour because it had been corrupted by radical feminism.

The court did affirm that 'signs of force or the threat of force' — wounds, torn clothes, the presence of a weapon — were not necessary to prove rape. This affirmation accords with the real-life fact that the amount of force necessary to achieve penetration is not much. But it is not true that the court opened the door to rape convictions in the kinds of cases Roiphe takes for the date-rape norm: sex in which the woman says yes but means no, or says yes, means yes, but regrets it later. The court said that consent, which need not be verbal, must be obtained for intercourse. It's easy to parody this view, as the defence counsel did with her joke about a 'consent form' — but all that it really means is that a man cannot penetrate a woman without some kind of go-ahead. Roiphe ridicules this notion as 'politically correct' and objects to educational materials that remind men that 'hearing a clear sober "yes" to the question "Do you want to make love?" is very different from thinking, "Well, she didn't say no." ' But is that such terrible advice? Roiphe herself says she wants women to be more vocal about sex, yet here she is dismissive of the suggestion that men ought to listen to them.

Roiphe's attemps to debunk statistics on the frequency of rape is similarly ill-informed. A substantial body of research, by no means all of it conducted by feminists, or even by women, supports the contention that there is a staggering amount of rape and attempted rape in the United States, and that most incidents are not reported to the police — especially when, as is usually the case, victim and offender know each other. For example, the National Women's Study, conducted by the Crime Victims Research and Treatment Center at the Medical University of South Carolina, working under a grant from the National Institute of Drug Abuse, which released its results last year, found that 13 per cent of adult American women – one in eight – have been raped at least once, 75 per cent by someone they knew. (The study used the conservative legal definition of rape which Roiphe favours: 'an event that occurred without the woman's consent, involved the use of force or threat of force, and involved sexual penetration of the victim's vagina, mouth or rectum.') Other researchers come up with similar numbers or even higher ones, and are supported by studies querying men about their own behaviour: in one such study, 15 per cent of the college men sampled said they had used force at least once to obtain intercourse.

Roiphe does not even acknowledge the existence of this sizable body of work – and it seems she hasn't spent much time studying the scholarly journals in which it appears. Instead, she concentrates on a single 1985 article in *Ms* magazine, which presented a preliminary journalistic account of an acquaintance-rape study conducted by Dr Mary Koss, a clinical psychologist now at the University of Arizona. Relying on opinion pieces by Neil Gilbert, a professor of social welfare at Berkeley, Roiphe accuses Koss of inflating her findings – one in eight students raped, one in four the victims of rape or attempted rape – by including as victims women who did not describe their experience as rape, although it met a widely accepted legal definition. It is unclear what Roiphe's point is – that women don't mind being physically forced to have sex as long as no one tells them it's rape? Surely she would not argue that the victims of other injustices – fraud, malpractice, job discrimination – have suffered no wrong as long as they are unaware of the law. Roiphe also accuses Koss of upping her numbers by asking respondents if they had ever had sex when they didn't want to because a man gave them alcohol or drugs. 'Why aren't college women responsible for their own intake of alcohol or drugs?' Roiphe asks, and it may be fair to say that the alcohol question in the study is ambiguously worded. But it's worth noting that the question doesn't come out of feminist fantasyland. It's keyed to a legal definition of rape which in many states includes sex obtained by intentional incapacitation of the victim with intoxicants – the scenario envisioned by my father. Be that as it may, what happens to Koss's figures if the alcohol question is dropped? The number of college women who have been victims of rape or attempted rape drops from one in four to one in five.

One in five, one in eight – what if it's 'only' one in ten or twelve? Social science isn't physics. Exact numbers are important, and elusive, but surely what is significant here is that lots of different studies, with different agendas, sample populations and methods, tend in the same direction. Rather than grapple with these inconvenient data, Roiphe retreats to her own impressions: 'If I was really standing in the middle of an epidemic, a crisis, if 25 per cent of my female friends were really being raped, wouldn't I know about it?' (Roiphe forgets that the one-in-four figure includes attempts, but let that pass.) As an experiment, I applied Roiphe's anecdotal method to myself, and wrote down what I knew about my own circle of acquaintance: eight rapes by strangers (including one on a college campus, two sexual assaults (one Central Park, one Prospect Park), one abduction (woman walking down street forced into car full of men), one date rape involving a Mickey Finn, which resulted in pregnancy and abortion, and two stalkings (one ex-lover, one deranged fan); plus one brutal beating by a boyfriend, three incidents of childhood incest (none involving therapist-aided 'recovered memories'), and one bizarre incident in which a friend went to a man's apartment after meeting him at a party and was forced by him to spend the night under the shower, naked, while he debated whether to kill her, rape her or let her go. The most interesting thing about this tally, however, is that when I mentioned it to a friend he was astonished – he himself knew of only one rape victim in his circle, he said – but he knows several of the women on my list.

It may be that Roiphe's friends have nothing to tell her. Or it may be that they have nothing to tell *her*. With her adolescent certainty that bad things don't happen, or that they happen only to weaklings, she is not likely to be on the receiving end of many painful, intimate confessions. The one time a fellow-student tells her about being raped (at knife-point, so it counts), Roiphe cringes like a high-school veg-etarian dissecting her first frog: 'I was startled . . . I felt terrible for her. I felt like there was nothing I could say.' Confronted with someone whose testimony she can't dismiss or satirize, Roiphe goes blank.

Roiphe is right to point out that cultural attitudes towards rape, harassment, coercion and consent are slowly shifting. It is certainly true that many women today, most of whom would not describe themselves as feminists, feel outraged by male behaviour that previous generations – or even those women themselves not so long ago – quietly accepted as 'everyday experience'. Roiphe may even be right to argue that it muddies the waters when women colloquially speak of 'rape' in referring to sex that is caddish or is obtained through verbal or emotional pressure or manipulation, or when they label as 'harassment' the occasional leer or off-colour com-ment. But if we lay these terms aside we still have to account for the phenomenon they point to: that women in great numbers – by no means all on elite campuses, by no means all young – feel angry at and exploited by behaviour that many men assume is within bounds and no big deal. Like many of those men, Roiphe would like to short-circuit this larger discussion, as if everything that doesn't meet the legal defi-nition of crime were trivial, and any objection to it mere paranoia. For her, sex is basically a boys' game, with boys' rules, like football, and if a girl wants to make the team – whether by 'embracing experience' in bed or by attending a formerly all-male college – she has to play along and risk taking some knocks. But why can't women change the game, and add a few rules of their own? What's so 'utopian' about expecting men to act as though there are two people in bed and two sexes in the classroom and the workplace?

Roiphe gives no consistent answer to this question. Some-times she dismisses the problems as inconsequential: coerced intercourse is bad sex, widespread sexual violence a myth.

Sometimes she suggests that the problem is real, but is women's fault: they should be more feisty and vociferous, be more like her and her friends, one of whom she praises for dumping a glass of milk on a boy who grabbed her breast. (Here, in a typical muddle, Roiphe's endorsement of assertive behaviour echoes the advice of the anti-rape educational materials she excoriates.) Sometimes she argues that the women's movement has been so successful in moving women into the professions that today's feminists are whining about nothing. And sometimes she argues that men, if seriously challenged to change their ways and habits, will respond with a backlash, keeping women students at arm's length out of a fear of lawsuits, retreating into anxious nerdhood, like her male-feminist classmates, or even, like the male protagonist of David Mamet's *Oleanna*, becoming violent: 'Feminists, Mamet warns, will conjure up the sexist beast if they push far enough.'

Coming from a self-proclaimed bad girl and sexual rebel, this last bit of counsel is particularly fainthearted: now who's warning women about the dangers of provoking the savage male? When Roiphe posits a split between her mother's generation of feminists – women eager to enter the world and seize sexual freedom – and those of today, who emphasise the difficulties of doing either, she has it wrong, and not just historically. (Sexual violence was a major theme of seventies feminism, in whose consciousness-raising sessions women first realised that rape was something many of them had in common.) The point she misses is that it was not the theories of academics or of would-be Victorian maidens masquerading as Madonna fans that made sexual violence and harassment an issue. It was the movement of women into male-dominated venues – universities, professions, blue-collar trades – in sufficiently great numbers to demand real accommodation from men both at work and in private life. If Roiphe's contention that focusing on 'victimhood' reduces women to passivity were right, the experience of Anita Hill would have sent feminists off weeping, *en masse*, to a separatist commune. Instead, it sparked a wave of activism that revitalised street-level feminism and swept unprecedented numbers of women into Congress.

Roiphe is so intent on demonizing the anti-rape movement that she misses an opportunity to address a real deficiency of much contemporary feminism. The problem isn't that acknowledging women's frequent victimisation saps their get-up-and-go and allows them to be frail flowers; it's that the discourse about sexuality says so little about female pleasure. Unfortunately, Roiphe, too, is silent on this subject. We hear a lot about heavy drinking, late nights, parties, waking up in strange beds, but we don't hear what made those experiences worth having, except as acts of rebellion. In a revealing anecdote, she cites with approval a friend who tells off obscene phone callers by informing them that she was her high school's 'blow job queen'. Not to detract from that achievement, but one wonders at the unexamined equation of sexual service and sexual selfhood. Do campus bad girls still define their prowess by male orgasms rather than their own?

It's sad for Roiphe and her classmates that they are coming of age sexually at a time when sex seems more fraught with danger and anxiety than ever. Indeed, Aids is the uneasily acknowledged spectre hovering over *The Morning After*: the condom, not the imaginary consent form, is what really put a damper on the campus sex scene. Certainly Aids gives new urgency to the feminist campaign for female sexual self-determination, and has probably done a lot, at both conscious and unconscious levels, to frame that quest in negative rather than positive terms. But that's just the way we live now – and not only on campus. Rape, coercion, harassment, the man who edits his sexual history and thinks safe sex kills passion, the obscene phone call that is no longer amusing because you're not in the dorm anymore but living by yourself in a not-so-safe neighbourhood and it's three in the morning: it's not very hard to understand why women sometimes sound rather grim about relations between the sexes.

It would be wonderful to hear more from women who are none the less 'embracing experience', retaining the vital spark of sexual adventure. Roiphe prefers to stick to the oldest put-down of all: Problems? What problems? It's all in your head.

From *Reasonable Creatures: Essays on Women and Feminism*, published by Vintage.

# MARGERY BREWS

*Letters from Margery Brews to John Paston III*

1477, February

Right reverend and worshipful and my right well-beloved
Valentine, I recommend me unto you full heartily, desiring
to hear of your welfare, which I beseech Almighty God
long for to preserve unto his pleasure and your heart's
desire. And if it please you to hear of my welfare, I am not
in good heal of body nor of heart, nor shall be till I hear
from you;

> For there wots no creature what pain that I endure,
> And for to be dead, I dare it not discure.

And my lady my mother hath laboured the matter to my
father full diligently, but she can no more get than ye know
of, for the which God knoweth I am full sorry.

But if that ye love me, as I trust verily that ye do, ye will
not leave me therefor; for if that ye had not half the live-
lode that ye have, for to do the greatest labour that any
woman alive might, I would not forsake you.

> And if ye command me to keep me true wherever I go,
> Iwis I will do all my might you to love and never no
>     mo.
> And if my friends say that I do amiss, they shall not
>     me let so for to do,
> Mine heart me bids evermore to love you
> Truly over all earthly thing,
> And if they be never so wroth, I trust it shall be
>     better in time coming.

No more to you at this time, but the Holy Trinity have you in keeping. And I beseech you that this bill be not seen of none earthly creature save only yourself, &c. And this letter was indite at Topcroft with full heavy heart, &c.[1]

By your own M. B.

1477, February

Right worshipful and well–beloved Valentine, in my most humble wise I recommend me unto you, &c. And heartily I thank you for the letter which that ye sent me by John Beckerton, whereby I understand and know that ye be purposed to come to Topcroft in short time, and without any errand or matter but only to have a conclusion of the matter betwixt my father and you. I would be most glad of any creature alive so that the matter might grow to effect. And there as ye say, an ye come and find the matter no more toward than ye did aforetime ye would no more put my father and my lady my mother to no cost nor business for that cause a good while after, which causeth mine heart to be full heavy; and if that ye come and the matter take to none effect, then should I be much more sorry and full of heaviness.

And as for myself, I have done and understand in the matter that I can or may, as God knoweth. And I let you plainly understand that my father will no more money part withal in that behalf but £100 and 50 mark, which is right far fro the accomplishment of your desire. Wherefore, if that ye could be content with that good, and my poor person, I would be the merriest maiden on ground. And if ye think not yourself so satisfied, or that ye might have much more good, as I have understand by you afore, good, true, and loving Valentine, that ye take no such labour upon you as to come more for that matter; but let i(t) pass, and never more to be spoken of, as I may be your true lover and bedewoman during my life.

[1] It was written by her father's clerk, Thomas Kela.

No more unto you at this time, but Almighty Jesus preserve you both body and soul, &c.

By your Valentine, Margery Brews

From *The Paston Letters*, edited by Norman Davies, published by Oxford University Press.

# CLARA PIRIZ
*Marriage by Pros and Cons*

Written to her husband whilst she was in exile in Holland, this letter was Clara Piriz's first uncensored communication with him. He had been a political prisoner in Uruguay for twelve years.

*Abcoude, Holland,*
*May 12, 1984*

Dear Kiddo,

I am writing this letter with no margins, without counting lines, or pages, without measuring my words a damn bit. Our first communication uncensored and uncut.

The big question is if I will manage to write without self-censorship . . . internalised censorship. Fear. My fear of causing you pain, of showing myself as I am, of confusing you in my confusion . . . My fear of losing what I've gained and gaining what I've lost . . .

A while ago I wrote you that it would be good for you to try to get out with a passport that would allow you to come and go. Let me explain why. At bottom it just has to do with another fear: the fear of ruining your life . . . even more.

Living in exile is a bitch. 'Sure,' you say, 'it can't be worse than prison.' True, prison is much worse. But, there is one fundamental difference: In prison you have to use all your energy to survive in a situation that doesn't depend on you and that you can't change. To survive in exile you have to use all your energy to change a situation of terrible inertia and, if it changes, it will be only because of your personal effort.

You arrive here with nothing, no friends, no job, no

*35*

house, no family. You don't understand the system in which you've somehow got to function. The place assigned to you is marginal, socially, economically, politically, culturally, emotionally. No one gives a damn about you. You have no history. Or rather, the history you have, no one cares about. Although suddenly it occurs to some reporter to use you as material for an article. A monkey in the zoo. And you accept, of course, because it's part of the political work: call attention to Uruguay, get political pressure. But if you achieve anything, no one cares. There are too many people. Most of all there are too many foreigners. Discrimination exists and it is rough. It sucks to feel looked down on, it sucks to have to do twice as much to get credit for half. It sucks when you say something and they look at you: '*and where did you crawl out . . .*' Not to mention worse things, like insults and violence.

But not all of it comes from outside of us; a lot we bring on ourselves. Most of the exiles resist adapting. They don't want to be here; they didn't choose to come to this country; everything is going wrong for them. The Dutch 'smell bad'; '*you know how they are.*' The exiles don't want to learn this fucking language, they refuse to give two and be counted for one. '*What for, anyway, if I'm going to leave . . .*' Result: Many of them have ended up completely screwed. Ten years of doing nothing of any worth, always running around, drinking beer and Geneva gin. Some of them read a lot, they remind me of your brother, a vagabond with books under his arm. Others have made a way for themselves, working like mules. Some have had the advantage of having studied, others of being stubborn workers with the 'nasty habit of earning their living.' This small group has one other problem: We are isolated because there's not enough time and energy to work, learn the language, etc . . . and still maintain friendships scattered all around the country.

A while ago I was talking with two Chileans and an Argentine woman I see regularly (a recently found remedy for the isolation). They said that even though they work, speak Dutch and have Dutch friends, communication with them had a limit they couldn't cross. I've heard that from other people. I must confess that is not the case with me. I have good friends who are Dutch, with whom my communication is excellent.

Well, as you see I'm not painting you a very pleasant picture. I can imagine that after twelve years in jail all this seems banal, but experience shows that once you are here the twelve years of jail don't help you think, '*What a terrific time I'm having.*' On the contrary, those years are one more problem.

In your case, there might be some points in your favour. Supposing our relationship works out (another subject altogether), I have made a way that can make your adjustment easier.

You might ask yourself if I am telling you this to try to discourage you. No. What it means is that I know what you'll have to face if you come here. And I don't want to have it on my conscience that I lured you with a siren song.

Our situation is not very encouraging either: two years of living together in very abnormal conditions. Twelve years without seeing each other: you in jail, which has certainly changed you. Neither one of us knows what problems are going to crop up from that. Certainly, within normal limits, you've changed a great deal. But it's also logical to expect less normal changes. There is no superman who can come unscathed out of one of those places. I don't believe those people – and there are some – who come out saying, '*Prison? A great experience, it's nothing.*' I also have lived through very hard experiences; I also am very much marked.

Besides, as a couple we're going to face a very strange situation. I have matured in this country, I have carried out a whole process of learning, of critical integration, of getting situated here, which you, one way or another, will have to carry out. This puts you in a position of dependence on me, which does not contribute to a healthy adult emotional relationship.

I'm finishing this letter today, June 24. Happy birthday! After yesterday's phone conversation I have such anxiety to see you, to talk to you, to touch you, that I can't imagine how I'm going to live from now until we see each other.

Yet there's so much we will have to discuss and go through!

And don't get all romantic on me and tell me that love, or the will to love, can overcome everything. No. It can overcome a lot, it is an essential condition, but not enough. I've seen so many who could not withstand the pressures of the change.

From a very young age, I have been bothered by rules without reasons, by *just because* or *because I said so* or *because that's the way it has to be*. It has bothered me as much in my social as in my private life. And systematically I have created a new set of rules based on my own experiences, on their analysis and synthesis and also on the reading and studies of the ideas of other (wiser) people. This attitude toward life is not new for me. Just think, if not, Carolina would not exist. Carolina was not an impulse, a mistake, a transgression. For me she was a conscious moral act which I have never regretted.

It was not always so easy: For years I struggled inside myself. Because sincerity is one of my values, at times I had to choose between the risk of destroying you or lying in the gentle way, by keeping quiet. Sometimes I kept quiet, sometimes I didn't. Finally I arrived at a formula: I'd try to let you know as best as possible how I felt about a lot of things and avoid the details that could be painful for you.

But my evolution is not only in that area. Most important to me is my maturity and my independence. That's why I made that comment on the phone yesterday: 'You are going to have a hard time with me.' I don't like to be ordered around, or told what to do. I reaffirm my right to my own decisions, your right to your own decisions, our right to be and think differently.

When I stayed alone with the girls I had to perform all of the roles; I was their mother and their father and their pet dog, too. I got used to it and from there I chose what I liked best to do, and that's not necessarily the womanly duties. Therefore (referring to a fantasy you wrote me about that frightened me): If you want homemade ravioli, make them yourself. I'll help you eat them. And I'll drink the wine. As a housekeeper I am consciously a disaster. My work is much more important to me, and my personal and professional development more than anything. For years my possibilities were limited by the urgency of moment to moment life, and by the girls' ages. Never the less, I got started with a brave effort. Now they are grown, they have their own independence, they're not attached to me, and I have found a phenomenal job. You can imagine that I'm grabbing on to that with all my strength. At my age it's my last chance and I can't and don't want to miss it.

We don't know what each of us means by a 'primary relationship.' You said it very blithely, as if there was a universally accepted formula. But I am certain that it's not that way. When I was twenty years old, I believed it, but not now, and that is not disillusionment, not at all, it's wisdom.

For instance, you asked me if I had a boyfriend. You didn't know how to deal with my answer. You said that could surely be the biggest stumbling block, and I answer you that the stumbling block is not that he exists . . . but the fact that *I* am capable of having a boyfriend.

I hold that I have been relentlessly faithful. Perhaps not in the way that you mean, but I'd bet if we talked about it, you'd see my way is much better.

Why do I want to see you? Because I do. Because I also allow myself the right to be (every once in a while) compulsive. I'm doing fine, I have a good job, a good social life, a serene and comforting relationship, the girls are growing up with no problems. Then why create problems for myself? Why not leave things as they are? Because I want to see you. Because I would feel terribly frustrated not to see you, because it would be a lack of respect for you, for me, for what we were, for what we are, and perhaps for what we might become . . . Because I want a second chance. Because only you and I can decide if it'll work or not. That decision is not for time, or distance, much less for the military to take. It's ours.

On the phone I found it hard to say I love you, for fear you misunderstood what I felt. So, I'll say: In my own way I love you. We'll have to see if my way and yours will meet – and grow.

Bye,
Clara

From *You Can't Drown the Fire: Latin American Women Writing in Exile*, edited by Alicia Partnoy, translated by Regina M Kreger, published by Virago.

# MARIE

## From *Women Like Us*

I didn't call myself a lesbian until about ten years ago, but I've had relationships with women for years and years. When I was twenty-one I had an affair with a woman and that was back in the West Indies, but we didn't have a word for what went on between us. We were good friends and sometimes shared the same bed, and it just happened without our really talking about it. We just reached out and touched. It was one of those things that happened. It felt okay to me, and it was the first really grown up experience I'd had. It just went on happening, and lasted for about a year, until I came to England. I left Barbados nearly thirty years ago, and the word 'lesbian' wasn't used there then. They were called 'Wicca'. It wasn't until I had been in England for several years that I heard the word 'lesbian'.

I came here to work because there was a lot of unemployment in Barbados and I couldn't find a job that paid a decent wage. At that time, I kept the house and did the cooking at home and worked as a dressmaker, but I was getting fed up with that and with not earning very much. I went to the employment agency to sign on and they said, 'Where do you want to work, here or abroad?' and I said, 'Anywhere.' At that time there was a big recruitment for England. A few weeks went by and I was interviewed to come to England to work for London Transport in 1960. I was nearly twenty-two years old.

I worked in a bus garage and was busy learning the job and settling in, but it was lonely. I had no family here, but a lot of boys from home came over to work in the garages, so I used to meet people I knew that way. Life was very tough for me, but I don't regret coming here, not really. It's all experience. I was here twelve years before I could afford to go home.

I've always been attracted to women, but it was very difficult to make contact, and I didn't hear about lesbians until many years after I arrived here. When I first came to England I didn't know where to go and meet people anyway. Also, there was a lot of racial prejudice for me to cope with, and I didn't get to meet many white women. But it was also difficult to meet other Black women, because most of them were married or in relationships with men. I think that at that time it was very difficult for white women to be out as lesbians, but for Black women it was difficult even to be single and independent. I was lonely and eventually I started relationships with men.

I had my next relationship with a woman in 1968, and again it just sort of 'happened'. She was married and after a while went back to her husband. I had two children by this time, and I was bringing them up on my own which was a real struggle, believe me, but they are grown up now, and I'm proud of them.

Then I had a relationship with a man on and off for ten years. But I did realise I had this attraction for women and I used to think 'What's wrong with you, girl?' I didn't tell anyone, it was all happening inside of me. I was struggling with my sexuality for three or four years, before I did anything about it. I'd been trying to work it out but didn't know where to go, what to do, how to meet other women. I was in my thirties then, and I just struggled on. More and more I began to think that I'm sure I fancy women and was beginning not to want this man around with whom I was having a relationship. I was working with this woman and we became really friendly. She was having problems with her husband, and she used to talk to me about it, and come to cry on my shoulder. We'd talk about everything, really — sex, lesbians, gays, everything, you know. It was the sort of friendship where you could talk about anything, and gradually I realised that I was falling in love with her. I thought, 'Oh, God, what do I do about this?' I was teaching her the book side of the job, and she'd come into my office every afternoon, and our chairs would be close together and our legs would touch, and

I'd get to the point where I'd have to walk out. It got really bad and I'd come home and try to work it out and think this is really desperate. But she was the type I could talk to about it, even though I knew nothing would come of it. I could tell her about it somehow and I worked out what to say. The next day, I said, 'Something really awful's happened.' And she started guessing all these things and she said, 'Are you in love with someone?' And I said, 'Yes, but it can't be, it's impossible.' And she started going through all my friends that she'd heard me mention saying things like 'Is it your friend's husband?' and, because we'd talked about lesbians and sexuality and all that, I said, 'It's a woman.' 'Oh well,' she said, 'if that's the way you feel.' And she accepted it. So she said, 'Well, who is it? Can't you tell her or stop seeing her or something?' And I said, 'It won't work out, it's impossible because she doesn't feel the same way,' and stuff like that. And she said, 'Well, stop seeing her.' So I said 'Okay, then, get out of my bloody office.' And she gave me a great big hug and a kiss and we just talked about it. But she understood. I just had to get it out of my system and it was really good after that, because she knew we could be okay about it. And we're still friends now.

My daughters were very good at sport and belonged to an athletics club. I became a very active committee member. I met a woman there, who was also involved in athletics, and we got to know each other quite well. She was someone I could talk to about the conflicts I was having about my sexuality. And then I saw these programmes on television about gays and lesbians, and somebody had sent in a letter in which she said that she liked men but kept having these feelings for women. I cut it out and kept it because I thought, 'That's me, that's just how I feel.' When my friend came round, I showed it to her. We talked about it and also about my feelings for my friend at work and she hugged me and said, 'You poor thing, what you must have been going through!' And we became really good friends. She said, 'There's nothing wrong with it – do something about it.' So I bought *Gay News* and looked at the clubs and started going there. At first, I was a bit nervous, because I walked into

*Sappho*[1] on my own and also this club, The Aztec, on my own. It was hard and I wouldn't do it now, but I was just desperate to meet other lesbians. After a while it was okay, and I met lots of people and made friends.

Before I was a lesbian, I wasn't sure what feminism was, but as a one-parent family I've always been strong and supported women's rights. As a lesbian, I became more politically aware and going to the Older Lesbian Network[2] (OLN) has helped. I just wish I could meet more older Black lesbians. I met three or four at the Black Lesbian Conference, but I suppose they have their lives sorted out and don't need organisations like the OLN which is all white, but I do; so I go.

At discos and other events that I go to, there are lots of young Black lesbians, but very young. I met a lot at the conference and we chat when I see them around, but I don't socialise much with them because of the age difference. I am proud to be an older Black lesbian, but I don't know many others. I am sure that there must be many in London, and I just wish I knew how we could contact each other.

I'd like to come out to all my friends and relatives, but I know there'd be problems. When the stuff about Martina (Navratilova) being a lesbian came out and my sister-in-law was talking about it, I said, 'Well, that's the way she is.' And my sister-in-law said, 'But it's wrong in God's eye. The Bible thing and all that. It's not natural, you know.' And I thought, 'Oh, God, here we go.' I felt that I would never be able to come out to my family. Coming out at work is difficult, because you're the same person you were yesterday, but to them you're somebody different. I don't really know what their reaction would be if they found out that I am a lesbian. I haven't really discussed it with them, but on the other hand, I haven't actually hidden it from them. I mean, I talk quite openly about my friendships with women and about my social life.

---

From *Women Like Us: Lives of Older Lesbians*, edited by Suzanne Neild and Rosalind Pearson, published by The Women's Press.

# LIV ULLMANN
## From *Changing*

Here Liv Ullmann is writing about her love affair with Ingmar Bergman.

It is a short love story that resembles so many others.

It lasted five years.

When she had lived with him for a few years she began to observe him. She would sit quietly and experience him as an individual.

One who no longer existed only in relation to her.

Gradually, within her an understanding of him awakened. The more he retreated from her, the better she understood him – as if the distance gave her clarity.

The fear diminished and the loneliness was easier to bear when she saw his insecurity.

She would become filled with tenderness and look beyond his violence and his injustice.

She was no longer blind to his faults and weaknesses, as she had been at the beginning. But her understanding and respect for him grew.

The adoration disappeared. She noticed that his hair was grey; he was much older than she; he was wise and stimulating; he was vain and egotistical.

And she discovered to her surprise that this was love.

With sadness she realised that it would soon be over, that she had come to him when he was already on his way somewhere else.

She looked at their child and realised that she would soon have that responsibility alone.

The last year she fought for their relationship, even though she knew it was hopeless, and not right for either of them.

And when it was all over she hoped that he would not be alone.

That the new woman would take better care of him than she had.

But of course it took her some time to reach that point.

She tried to recall who she had been when she came to the island five years before.

Something had been crushed in her, and something was more alive.

She had undergone a change.

And when bitterness and hate and despair were gone, she was sure she had experienced love and been enriched.

But she would never be able to talk about it.

She had seen into another person and was full of tenderness for what she had found.

For a period of time they had taken each other's hands and been painfully connected.

But only when it was all over did they become true friends.

From *Changing*, published by Weidenfeld & Nicholson Ltd.

# DIANNE LINDEN
## *In the Bleak Midwinter*

I fell in love with a baritone at the Pro Coro Christmas Concert last year: stayed in love with him for at least ten minutes because of his face. He bore the burden of homeliness, and I wanted to share it with him. I saw he had poor posture, thin shoulders, a slight paunch and that made me love him more. I was sure his appearance was caused by some difficulty in his life which could have been prevented by the love of a good woman, like me.

He had a real hangdog face: the kind of face that would look morosely at me over the breakfast table because the newspaper had gotten a little wet when it lay out on the porch steps in the snow, or because the three-minute egg I cooked him was really a seven. (Let's say I was thinking about knitting a new silver hat or a cobwebby pair of wings or a black, sequinned hat band, tasteful, in case someone I knew died and I had to go to the funeral: and I lost track of time.) He'd look at me over the newspaper, and I'd feel his disappointment that my control over time and the world in general was less significant than he'd expected.

He and I had never spoken, never looked deeply into each other's eyes, sighed, searched each other's mouths with tongues as eager to communicate as newly uncapped pens, yet I can say with sad certainty that if we were to meet and become lovers, one day his eyes would complain to me of my imperfections over the newspaper at breakfast, which I hardly ever eat, and I would have to ask him to leave.

He'd probably have brought two or three pipes with him to keep by the chair my cat slept in before he moved in with us on non-concert evenings: maybe a second tuxedo in case his awful need of me made it necessary for us to be together just before he went off to sing. He'd have shaving things, of course: a mug of soap, an old badger-hair shaving brush, a silver-handled razor engraved with someone else's initials, hair tonic, silk shorts: all those frugal accoutrements a man brings along with him when he means to stay a while, and I'd have to ask him to leave. (He would have left me anyway, when the next potentially omnipotent person came along.) I wouldn't like asking him to go. But I'd do it anyway.

It would be traumatic for me, watching him walk out of my door with his threadbare carpet bags, and wait on the porch for a taxi cab he probably couldn't afford, so instead of sending him a little note at the end of the concert saying, 'I loved your small, modest solo at the end of the Schütz piece. I was the tall woman in the purple parka who waved at you repeatedly from the front row. My name is Dianne. Please phone me at 455–6693 if you feel as lonely and nostalgic over Christmas as I do,' I put my boots on and went out for a caesar salad with a friend of mine who's gay. He already knows I'm not in control of anything much, and he apparently doesn't care.

From *Eating Apples: Knowing Women's Lives*, edited by Caterina Edwards and Kay Stewart, published by NeWest Press.

# CAROLE
*Interview with Debra*

Debra worked in prostitution for nine years. She is thirty-two years old and is presently working as a paralegal.

*Carole:* Where did you grow up?
*Debra:* My mother had me in Louisiana. I never met my father. I have no desire to. He just wanted some pussy and my mother happened to be there. From what I understand he was a jackass. He was already married. My mother had me, didn't tell her parents and then gave me up for adoption. I was gone from my mother for nine months. But when she was getting the final papers for the adoption, she said, 'No.' Meanwhile she'd gotten pregnant again. She told me the reason she'd gotten pregnant a second time was that she'd gone through this birth, mine, and felt empty. Then she decided that she was going to have me, too. She went to court and to this day she cries when she talks about it. It was awful! They called her names in court.

My mother moved to Wisconsin. I lived with my grandmother, who is wonderful. I love my grandmother! But she was a product of her times and she lived in a very tight-knit German–Polish community in Milwaukee. She wanted to tell the neighbours that I was a foster child. My mother told her, 'She's my daughter and I will never renounce her again.' And she didn't. I've always loved my mother for that. Except when I was doing the prostitution. She had quite a problem with it: She tends to get religious. I'm not religious. I believe that a lot of religious beliefs are man-made myths to keep people down. I believe in some superior being, but not some blond man who walked the earth.

My mother married when she had two children – my sister and me. As far as I'm concerned, he's my real father. I mean it's not hard to take a dick and put it in a pussy. It doesn't mean anything. What motherhood and fatherhood mean to me is the actual bringing up of the children and the love you give them.

We moved to Madison, where we lived until I was in the sixth grade. My mother always said that she'd have twelve children – six boys and six girls – by the time she turned forty. And she had her twelfth child five days before turning forty. She loves children.

I had a lot of responsibilities when I was a child, I think, almost *too* much. I remember making my first turkey dinner when I was in sixth grade. I did the babysitting for all the kids. I was a real responsible child mostly because I didn't have a choice. It wasn't, 'Could you,' it was, 'Do this.' Then we moved further out. Really in the boonies. We bought an old farmhouse with one acre. It didn't have any heat upstairs so we had to sleep downstairs – ten of us in the same bed.

My father was an alcoholic until I was about seventeen or eighteen. A really severe alcoholic. It was real hard for him to show affection. I always thought he hated me. Then he quit drinking with AA, his whole person changed. He became a more gentle, caring and thinking man. I couldn't believe it. I used to waitress in a bar where he used to drink. It was one of the hardest things I remember doing – serving him liquor when I knew he had a problem with it. He was spending money and we were broke. I remember being a kid and being hungry. I mean, I remember cutting up onions so that my stomach wouldn't hurt. But my parents did the best they could. We always had some place to stay and shoes and we never starved. I think it taught me a lot.

I've been working outside the home since I was thirteen. I've done a lot of jobs. My first farm work, I picked cucumbers for eight hours a day. It's back-breaking labour. And you didn't get paid shit for it. We worked for Del Monte, the pickle people. The older I got, after I left home, I realised that other kids didn't have to do so much. It kind of freaked me out. It made me realise how much I did do.

*Carole:* How did you get involved in prostitution?

*Debra:* Well, I turned my first trick a long time before I actually turned out as a prostitute. I had been in college for a while and I was working as a cocktail waitress because my parents couldn't afford to give me any money. And there was this assemblyman. Assemblymen really made me see what politicians were about – I'm telling you – these men were disgusting. They were gross. But they run our state. The people in Washington are probably worse, and they're running the country! This one man, one night, seduced me. He was older, probably in his fifties, and I was eighteen. He knew that he shouldn't have been doing that. He was married. Anyway, he gave me crabs and I never saw him again except where I worked. He had had his conquest, so that was that. But then I decided that I wanted to be an assembly page. To do that I had to be sponsored by an assemblyman. That's when I first turned a trick. I went up to him and I said, 'I want you to sponsor me.' He looked in my face and he knew better than to deny me. He was a politician and he didn't want it to get out. I was using sex as a tool, although not consciously. I was sexually harassed as a page and left. But that's another story.

Later I went to art school. And graduated. I had a 3.6 average. I worked house painting. I've had a lot of different jobs. I've worked in canning factories, which is horrendous work. That's why prostitution was so nice for me. Because you got a lot of money. You didn't take harassment. You didn't allow it. You were in control of the situation. You know? If someone patted my bottom, I got money for it. They didn't expect it to be part of the job. Which is very basically what I was going through with a lot of the other jobs. Being told that I should be thankful for the job. Please kiss my ass and thank me for giving you this shit job. You know? And I was getting totally fed up with it. So I started prostitution and took to it immediately.

*Carole:* Where did you start working?

*Debra:* Here in California, in the Bay Area. I moved out here in 1976. I met some people who were into prostitution and I turned out in February 1977. I liked being an artist and I was a good commercial artist. But I walked downtown San Francisco for months and nobody would give me a job. Not only would they not give me a job, they wouldn't look at my portfolio. Because I didn't have the work experience they wanted me to have, they wouldn't give me a How-do-you-do. People are fairly rude in a large city.

I worked with a group of women and one man. Right away. Thank God! I learned how to protect myself and my body. Another woman stood behind me as I worked. I got tutored in how to be a prostitute. That's the only way. I turned out on University Avenue in Berkeley.

The man never came out. A black man and a white woman on the stroll just ain't cool. The police would have a heyday. He'd go to jail and I wouldn't. It's ludicrous the racism in this country. I learned about racism in the seventh grade because the kids at school thought I was Mexican – but I didn't really learn about it until I turned out. It's sick. I've just been reading some books and I realise that a lot of times in the course of history common people, decent people, have allowed fanatics to control the way the world is run, mainly because they didn't step in and stop it. Because they're not fanatics. You know what I mean? I think racism is becoming more definite in this country because people who think like I do, or think like you do, aren't saying, 'Hey, wait a minute, I'm not going for it.'

*Carole:* Debra, what kind of violent incidents took place in your work?

*Debra:* Well, first of all, when I turned a trick, I did it the way I wanted to. I was in control. I was the boss. I didn't allow tricks to touch my genitals and I fucked them in my hand. I had a certain way that I tricked and if they didn't want to trick that way they could leave.

The only two times somebody did something to me personally were right after I turned out. It happened two weeks in a row. The first month I turned out, I had my women friends with me but I was young and naive. When you ride with a trick you're in their territory. You have to take special precautions even if it's three minutes or three blocks away.

You have your own specific route that you take. When you get in the car, you search it – you look in the glovebox. You keep your hand on the door handle at all times. You make sure that the door opens and closes before you get in. You watch every move the trick makes. He keeps both of his hands on the steering wheel. If you tell him to take a right, and he doesn't you're out of the car.

The first time, I took this trick to the trick pad. It was evening time, probably 10 pm or 11 pm. He was a young guy. It was really busy at the trick pad. He didn't want to wait. I didn't know you don't ride back with a trick who hasn't dated. So, I'm driving back and I'm looking out the window and the guy put a knife to my throat. He took me off for three, four hours in the hills of Albany. I tried every move I knew. I mean I cried, I pretended I liked it. I finally talked him into getting a room so that we'd spend the night together. Finally! So, we rode back to Berkeley and I jumped out of the car and I told him that he better get the fuck out of there and he drove away with his door flapping. He'd raped me numerous times.

*Carole:* Wasn't it hard to get into a car again after that?

*Debra:* No, I knew that I'd done it wrong. It's a dangerous business and you have to protect yourself. You know, the thing that saves a ho is her sixth sense. Her sense of people. You have to make up your mind about people within minutes. You get to be really good at that. Our rule is if someone looks at you the wrong way, and says hello how you don't like it, no matter how much money he's offering you, leave it alone. Follow your first mind. You can look in someone's eyes and see compassion or humaneness or you can see meanness or violence. And it works.

It happened to me another time, though, shortly after. This guy had apparently been doing it to other women in San Francisco, but I was in the Berkeley stroll, so we hadn't gotten the word yet. 'Cause normally if one ho knows, she'll let the other hos know. 'Cause you protect each other. This white, middle-aged, respectable looking man took me off and we were driving to the same trick pad. He pulled out a gun and said, 'Bitch, you make a move and I'll blow your head off.' I broke his windshield and I broke his glasses. But he kept driving and I was raped. That was the last time, though. And I was a ho for nine years.

*Carole:* Did you ever report these incidents to the police?

*Debra:* I can't tell you the countless times I've heard police say that a prostitute can't be raped. It really upsets me. I think a lot of men believe that. It's totally ridiculous. I've had friends who've gotten hurt. After a while you stop telling the police. Their attitude is, 'Hey, that's part of your job.' Probably a lot of women believe that, too. Though I've had less of that attitude from women than men – the attitude that a prostitute is putting herself out there and that she deserves what she gets, whether it's rape or getting beaten up.

*Carole:* Did you make a lot of money?

*Debra:* Yes! We made *beaucoup* money! My attitude was that I was going to get what I wanted. For so many years I'd been abused, mainly by men. Face it, the people who ran the factories and the jobs were mostly men. I got sick of men doing that to me. I made between three and five hundred dollars a night and sometimes more. I lived better than I did in my life. It was a going joke – 'Feed Debbie.' I was really little then. There had been so many times that I hadn't eaten before so I ate like a horse. And I had furs, leathers, silks. We rented yachts for New Year's Eve. It was great! But it was fast money and fast money goes fast. We didn't just blow it, though, we invested it in real estate. Then the Feds took everything. But that's a whole other story.

From *Sex Work: Writings by Women in the Sex Industry*, edited by Frédérique Delacoste and Priscilla Alexander, published by Cleis Press.

# COLETTE

## From *Break of Day*

> *'Are you imagining, as you read me,*
> *that I'm portraying myself? Have*
> *patience: this is merely my model.'*

*Sir,*

    *You ask me to come and spend a week with you, which means I would be near my daughter, whom I adore. You who live with her know how rarely I see her, how much her presence delights me, and I'm touched that you should ask me to come and see her. All the same I'm not going to accept your kind invitation, for the time being at any rate. The reason is that my pink cactus is probably going to flower. It's a very rare plant I've been given, and I'm told that in our climate it flowers only once every four years. Now, I am already a very old woman, and if I went away when my pink cactus is about to flower, I am certain I shouldn't see it flower again.*

    *So I beg you, Sir, to accept my sincere thanks and my regrets, together with my kind regards.'*

This note, signed '*Sidonie Colette, née Landoy*', was written by my mother to one of my husbands, the second. A year later she died, at the age of seventy-seven.

Whenever I feel myself inferior to everything about me, threatened by my own mediocrity, frightened by the discovery that a muscle is losing its strength, a desire its power or a pain the keen edge of its bite, I can still hold up my head and say to myself: 'I am the daughter of the woman who wrote that letter – that letter and so many more that I have kept. This one tells me in ten lines that at the age of seventy-six she was planning journeys and undertaking them, but that waiting for the possible bursting into bloom of a tropical flower held everything up and silenced even her heart, made for love. I am the daughter of a woman who, in a mean, close-fisted, confined little place, opened her village home to stray cats, tramps and pregnant servant-girls. I am the daughter of a woman who many a time, when she was in despair at not having enough money for others, ran through the wind-whipped snow to cry from door to door, at the houses of the rich, that a child had just been born in a poverty-stricken home to parents whose feeble, empty hands had no swaddling clothes for it. Let me not forget that I am the daughter of a woman who bent her head, trembling, between the blades of a cactus, her wrinkled face full of ecstasy over the promise of a flower, a woman who herself never ceased to flower, untiringly, during three quarters of a century.'

Now that little by little I am beginning to age, and little by little taking on her likeness in the mirror, I wonder whether, if she were to return, she would recognise me for her daughter, in spite of the resemblance of our features. She might if she came back at break of day and found me up and alert in a sleeping world, awake as she used to be, and I often am, before everyone.

Before almost everyone, O my chaste, serene ghost! But you wouldn't find me in a blue apron with pockets full of grain for the fowls, nor with secateurs or a wooden pail. Up before almost everyone, but half-naked in a fluttering wrap hastily slipped on, standing at my door which had admitted a nightly visitor, my arms trembling with passion and shielding – let me hide myself for shame! – the shadow, the thin shadow of a man.

'Stand aside and let me see,' my beloved ghost would say. 'Why, isn't what you're embracing my pink cactus, that has survived me? How amazingly it's grown and changed! But now that I look into your face, my child, I recognise it. I recognise it by your agitation, by your air of waiting, by the devotion in your outspread hands, by the beating of your heart and your suppressed cry, by the growing daylight all about you, yes, I recognise, I lay claim to all of that. Stay where you are, don't hide, and may you both be left in peace, you and the man you're embracing, for I see that he is in truth my pink cactus, that has at last consented to flower.'

From *Break of Day*, translated by Enid Mcleod, published by Secker & Warburg Ltd.

# CAROL MARA
## *The Hardest Love*

When we go back into the room they have opened the blinds and we can see the stars and the lights from the town below us. Our son is lying on a bed now, the sheets straight and neat around his broken body. Beside his head there is a pale gold orchid translucent against the stark white sheet. He is holding the calico doll his sister has made in the hours just gone, her message inscribed on the back in felt pen –

> *Dear William,*
> *I will miss you so very much and I will love you forever.*
> *Catherine.*

On the front she has drawn a happy face with curly brown hair, purple shorts and a green shirt.

At the moment of his passing just an hour before, his father called out his name, over and over, wailing for his son. His older brother stood by his feet the tears rolling down his face, 'See ya, Will', the only words he can find to say goodbye, the words that passed between them every day. Catherine, her face red and swollen with tears and weariness clung more fiercely to my breast.

I look down at my beautiful son who has been stolen from me. I hold his familiar slender hand, I stroke his forehead, the small scar where he fell off his bike; I lay my hands along his freckled cheeks. What am I to do with this portion of love, enough to last a lifetime, I have stored in my heart? I can feel the pain already, sharp and bitter, as it struggles for release.

I am holding the hand of the baby I bore, the child I nurtured, the boy I cherished. His fingers stay curled around mine when I press them down. How can I leave this child of my heart? My warm tears fall on to his bare shoulders, I touch the drops, his skin is cool and I repeat the words I said five hours earlier when I first saw him, the machines whooshing, the blood seeping from his head, his eyes half open, a dull film over them, 'He's not there anymore.'

We just sit, touching and stroking and talking, telling him the things he always knew, how dearly we love him, the fine son and brother he is; how our hearts are breaking that he only had thirteen years to know the beauty, the wonder and the adventure of life, that we only had thirteen years in which to give our love and care to him.

Forever my son will be thirteen years old, he will not grow to be a man and the outrage of his death begins to envelope me: an unknown driver has run him down as he walked with friends beside the road. I have to fight to quell the anger; I want to stay with the love.

Sometime later we know we must leave him. I place the doll on his chest and press his hands around it. The doll, invested with so much love and love foregone will be forever with him on his journey to the farthest places.

# LUCY GOODISON

## Really Being in Love Means Wanting to Live in a Different World

So read a situationist leaflet in the heady days of the 1970s.[1] The Left and the women's movement have traditionally given 'falling in love' a very bad press. Women have pointed to the way it tends to make us feel helpless, passive, uncomprehending, dependent, immobilised: the very feelings we are struggling to leave behind. Radical political and social movements told us that 'falling in love' is individualistic, objectifying, linked to escapist notions of romantic love, exploited by advertisements to encourage consumerism, and tied firmly at the far end to the great institution of marriage which helps to keep the cogs of society ticking over. All in all we can see that it is clearly 'incorrect', and one reaction has been to ignore it.[2]

And yet falling in love does not go away. We all do it. It is gripping, exciting. We long for it. It makes other more politically 'correct' areas of our life pale by comparison. It keeps cropping up. Its power is unquestionable.

Perhaps somewhere between the traditional view of accepting it as an inevitable part of human nature, and the tendency to dismiss it as a capitalist con, there is a third path: one which involves looking at the experience in detail and grappling with its process. In this way we might gain more access to using its power rather than becoming its victim. This has not been done. As a subject it has largely remained untouchable. Perhaps we secretly like having an area of our lives that we cannot explain and are not expected to.

As with a religious experience, no one can contradict our feelings.[3] We are sent reeling into talk about 'wonderful feelings' which 'just happen'. We seem to fear that if we look too

hard its magic will vanish. We can however try to chart
unknown seas, not in order to plunder them, or cut them
down to size, but the better to explore and travel them. We
are not trying to reduce the excitement in our lives, but to
increase our ability to choose and direct that excitement.

So what is falling in love like? How does it happen? What
are the steps, the progressions? It is not one unitary or primary experience, but rather a number of experiences bound
up together, different feelings present in different people in
different proportions. It may vary as widely as one orgasm
from another. However, there are certain common experiences, and before investigating the 'whys' and 'wherefores' I
shall briefly sketch what these seem to be. From women's
accounts, some common threads seem to recur whether the
object of our passion is a man or a woman, so I shall describe
both together as different aspects of the same process. I shall
use women's novels, poems and personal accounts, as well as
some of the media clichés which have influenced us so
strongly and which remain the backdrop of our efforts to
create a new language for our experience.

Over the years I have done extensive field work on this
subject. I am not describing a place where I have not been,
though I have never written about it before. My account feels
very tentative, like early maps of uncharted territories, and
much of it is written in blood.

Step one, you find someone to love. It often happens
through 'love at first sight', the impact of a first encounter:

> Who is this stick of corn? or is she a lion?
> she's doing yoga on the lawn
> brown body bending like a snake
> her face is miles wide; she is open
> eyes welcome . . . have I really known her
> somewhere before? was I born with her?[4]

A bell rings, something beckons far beyond words. Yet often
the reason for the attraction is not obvious. The objects of
our passion often lack traditional 'qualities' like money or

looks. They may also be too old, too young. They may be different from us, unsuitable or unavailable. But the line is cast, the bait is taken, and we are hooked.

What happens next? One friend compared falling in love to LSD in the way it changes reality. Another woman writes that it is as if the world has been stopped and started again.[5] We often hear about a general sensation of disorientation, a feeling that the cosmos has moved in its tracks, the concrete and the clay beneath our feet have crumbled. And this shifting world is permeated by a terrible wanting. Marge Piercy, in her novel *Small Changes*, describes how Miriam experiences the power and relentlessness of this yearning:

> Where so much had been, plans and projects and curiosities and relationships and speculations and histories, was now everything and nothing in one: this painful hollow wanting, this fierce turbulence, this centring about him white hot and icy, cold and dark and bright.[6]

Miriam lies on her bed in embryo position curled round her obsession and feels as if her self and identity are dissolving. Her ability to operate in the world is seriously impaired. 'I can't do my homework and I can't think straight,' sang Connie Francis in my teens. Miriam has a more grown-up version of the same problem:

> When she did her work at all, she did it perfunctorily . . . she would resent the trivial chatter about programming languages that made her for a moment unable to loose her whole energies on her obsession . . . She seemed to have nothing left for anyone else, anything else. She was stupefied in general and in that one touch point intensely burning like a laser.[7]

Though the overwhelming feeling is of emotion or intensity, it is very localised and there can be a narrowing of vision, a deadening of other areas of life. Stored aggression erupts as violence; stored love, too, seems able to break out with an edge as cutting as a knife.

It is this laser-like cutting quality which can give being in love an active, rebellious, even political flavour. Sometimes there can be anger contained in that ferocious energy: a schoolteacher angry at the reactionary staff falls in love with a sixth-former; a teenager falls in love with someone who will shock her parents. It can be a way of cocking a snook at authority, of striking a blow at society. Traditionally, falling in love is a great defier of convention, breaking barriers imposed by class, race and prejudice: the lady of the manor who falls in love with the gypsy, the Capulet who falls for the Montague. It can act as the beam of light which cuts through the crap, which reveals the mediocrity, hypocrisy and banality of so much in our society. As the libertarian magazine *Ink* pointed out in their 'In Love' issue:

> The experience ... gives us a glimpse of the exuberance and energy which might be set free when our relations with one another are liberated from the system that perverts them ... Being in love shatters ... constraints. We give presents instead of buying and selling, we touch instead of avoiding one another's eyes.[8]

Amidst alienation it makes us feel inexorably connected; amidst deceit its sheer impact makes us feel that something is real; in muddy waters of pain and compromise it can feel like a lifeline. Though it can obliterate the rest of the world, sometimes it can also make the whole world come alive. Sometimes its light, rather than turning inwards, can turn outwards to infuse the whole range of vision. Something in it tells us it could be a revolutionary force: 'They never wanted us to feel like this. Killers beware! With love like this we can move mountains and break your prisons down. It is no dope to help us to forget, oh no. This love is dangerous.'[9]

Another contradiction with falling in love is that although we may feel vanished and drained into the loved one, we may also at some level feel ourselves more intensely. We are superconscious of something important happening to us. We step into the limelight in our own lives. There can even be an unwonted narcissism or relish in our experience. The strength of our feelings imparts a new self-confidence and meaning to life.[10] Though we are not in control of it, we are undoubtedly the carriers of some huge power:

> I have a feeling, a strange feeling:
> she seems to potentiate me. I am expanding: will I burst
> like a star on the world?[11]

Or as Marge Piercy describes it: 'Much of the time she felt lucky, chosen, exalted. Her life seemed infused with intensity, a plenum, shining and holy. She was never bored. Her previous life seemed vacuous by comparison.'[12]

How does this whole experience connect with romantic love? Romantic fantasies (about moonlit nights, wedding bells, true love to the death against all opposition, and so on) may be an important element, but from all accounts they are rarely central. They may be the preformed moulds which society offers us to pour our love into: but they are not its source. These fantasies are pretty, while the central drive of falling in love seems to be more of a blood-and-guts affair. It is not just glamorous and appealing. More than wanting to cosset the beloved, we may feel we want to eat them alive. We may idealise the loved one, but that may slip away like a mask to reveal ferocious hatred and rage if things go wrong. Romantic feelings and fantasies may be the blossoms produced by being in love, but its roots lie deeper in the earth. The power it feeds on is not essentially romantic, but one that tears at the innards.

So what is this strange and physically overwhelming power? Is it primarily sexual? Here comes another irony. In some of the most passionate accounts of 'being in love', the sexual experience itself is not totally satisfactory. Erica Jong writes in an autobiographical novel about a woman who leaves a very compatible sexual relationship with her husband for a love-affair in which at first she finds it very hard to reach orgasm:

> He fucked as if he wanted to get back inside the womb. My heart was beating so hard I couldn't come . . . Josh felt like kin to me, my long-lost brother . . . I went right to the edge of orgasm and wasn't able to come. This had happened the night before . . . And the oddest part of it was: I didn't care.
>
> We locked together like two pieces of a puzzle . . . What other point was there in bringing a man and woman together *except* to stretch the soul and expand the imagination, except to tear things apart and put them back together in new ways? . . . The mere rubbing that sooner or later results in orgasm was not all one looked for. A vibrator could do that.[13]

Here is another woman's experience:

> The sex was wonderful, overwhelming, not because it worked particularly well in itself, but because it was with him. One of my most most precious memories is of a night when I simply lay sleepless and blissed-out in his arms. What was most powerful was not the sex but the *intimacy* I felt with him.[14]

We hear accounts of passionate love where sex 'works' perfectly, or relationships which centre on the strong bonding of sex, but there are also accounts of sexual difficulties and incompatibilities which are dwarfed by the power of being in love. Some intense bonding seems to occur which may channel through sexuality, but is not subsumed in it. Pure lust is generally recognised as a different experience. It is possible to feel a magnificent lust for a person, to connect with her or him intensely and magically through sex, without ever feeling 'in love'. Sexual feelings may be an important factor in falling in love, but it is as if those feelings are informed from another source, from some other connection between the two people.

Finally, I need to mention how falling in love can end. Sometimes it endures, developing into a long-term relationship. What is then retained or lost of the original impetus is part of a wider discussion about long-term sexual relationships. Does the intensity of the passion fade, endure, transmute? Is it compatible with daily life, living together, children? What is the difference between 'falling in love', 'being in love', and 'loving' someone in a steadier and more whole way? These issues fall outside the scope of this piece. But perhaps more common than the happy-ever-after ending is for a relationship to die young. Apart from cases where circumstances tear lovers apart, this generally happens through one person 'falling out of love'.

Like falling in love, falling out of love can happen suddenly. You may wake up one morning and feel different. It can be as if a dream has passed to be replaced by reality. The person suddenly looks very ordinary. What did I see in her/him? Sometimes there is a sensation of relief at the return to 'normality'. Sometimes there is a vague sense of loss at the inexplicable passing of passion:

> Where are the sons of summer now?
> The winter has come
> And you don't know how to turn your dreams into
>   coal . . .
> And I can't help but get a little bit blue
> Thinking about the precious nothing we once knew.
>
> (Carly Simon)

A few nostalgic grains of stardust are left in hand, and life goes on as normal.

Alternatively, it happens the other way round. Some loves are unrequited from the start, or the other person may start to give you a hard time or fall out of love with you. Then comes more than a vague sense of loss. That is when the heartaches really begin. In *Small Changes* Miriam feels her strength and identity slip away:

> She waited. She waited two hours, while anger and resent-
> ment wound her tighter and tighter. She tried to fight her
> tension . . . Why must she sit like — like a woman was
> supposed to, stewing? Her anxiety stripped away her sense
> of herself as a strong person moving through things in her
> own style. She became dependent woman. She became
> scared woman. This waiting had teeth.[15]

Very recognisable is the process whereby Miriam becomes more and more desperate to regain the love that is slipping away from her. Our efforts to recover, to rebuild our power in ourselves, are continually dogged by referral to that other person who remains the magical standard by which every-thing is measured, the philosopher's stone without which nothing can be gold.

What is so excruciating about this state is its closeness to the worst stereotypes of how women are meant to be: dependent, empty, passive, waiting, pleading. However hard we fight it consciously, we can feel drawn to wallow in the 'rich stew of masochism'.[16] It hurts so *good*. We feel 'right', we feel in character, as if the pain is part of our birthright as women, so intimate and close that it almost becomes precious to us, as Marge Piercy writes of Janis Joplin:

> You embodied the pain hugged to the breasts like a baby.
> You embodied the beautiful blowsy gum of passivity . . .
> That willingness to hang on the meathook and call it love,
> That need for loving like a screaming hollow in the soul.[17]

When the beloved is completely and irrevocably lost, the immensity of love's joy can turn its flipside to reveal an immensity of pain. The craziness of happiness can come perilously near real craziness and self-hatred, as one woman writes:

The same waves that crested in the elation of BE HERE NOW and ALL IS ONE sucked me back under and I was CRAZY as never before. I lost control. I suffered disbelief and an excruciating desire not to BE ME that allowed me to touch bottom in some amorphous way ... and declare 'I am bankrupt'.[18]

This love that can be like a meathook, this love that can drive us crazy, where does its power come from? I have described the terrain, the superficial process, but what are the force fields at work under the earth? Like many major experiences, falling in love is perhaps over-determined and can be explained on a number of different levels. I shall mention some of these, and describe some of the factors which may conspire to send us hurtling over the abyss. I shall also mention various theoretical frameworks which may throw light on the process, drawing mainly but not exclusively on psychological models placed within the social context of capitalism. Knowing whether the same factors would be present or relevant in another culture or another period of history would illuminate our political understanding of falling in love, and our sense of how that experience could be transformed; but this question would need a separate article to do it justice, and here I can only bear it in mind.

One precipitating factor seems to be immediate life-circumstances, which often include some kind of 'rebound' situation, or a reaction to suppression. People often seem to fall in love as a reaction from another relationship. The original relationship may be deteriorating, or there may be unexpressed resentment in it, perhaps due to infidelity, neglect, or subtle domination by one partner. A certain level of need or tension has accumulated. Strong feelings are present but they are blocked or stuck. Then suddenly an outburst of passion shoots, not into hurt or anger in that relationship, but into overwhelming love for a different person. The new relationship allows a release of feeling and expression which had been blocked in the first relationship. The connection of the new passion to the original person is rarely felt; often s/he appears to be completely wiped off the map. Thus Erica Jong's heroine reacts with total blankness to the husband she has just left: 'Couldn't he hear in my voice that I didn't miss him at all, that he had never even existed, that he was a ghost, a shadow? I suppose not.'[19] This view of falling in love presents it as a substitution, its fierce energy partly fuelled by the need to escape from an existing situation.

Sometimes that situation does not involve another person. Sometimes it is simply a long period in an emotional desert, a long period without joy or sexual satisfaction or physical affection or expression or intensity in any relationship or activity, which builds up until there is a 'charge' of need which will eventually spark across to make contact with another person. Is this level of repression, in relationships and outside them, a feature specific to capitalism? *Ink* suggested that even in a Utopia we might need 'release in concentrated bursts of energy. Would communal, ecstatic, religious, spiritual, sexual experiences be a feasible alternative?'[20] However the charge builds up, that charge and the readiness to fall in love lie in the subject. She may even make a false start and have a short-lived infatuation with one person before falling deeply in love with another: a kind of practice run. Her antennae are out. Falling in love is what she needs. The timing is hers.

But how do we choose the object of so much unstinting affection? What qualifies them for the job? One theory proposed by various schools of psychology is that they fill gaps in ourselves, resonating with qualities which are absent or not fully realised in our own personality. This means we love not the whole, but only that part of the person which we need to complete us. As Fritz Perls of the Gestalt school of therapy put it:

We don't usually love a *person* That's very, very rare. We love a certain *property* in that person, which is either identical with our behaviour or supplementing our behaviour, usually something that is a supplement to us. We think we are in love with the total person, and actually we are disgusted with other aspects of this person.[21]

So what kind of properties do we love in the beloved? Often it is something which is forbidden in ourselves, perhaps something quite different or alien, and this is why the chosen one may at first sight appear very unsuitable. S/he expresses qualities we have buried in ourselves, whether they are painfully unacceptable or idealised.[22] According to humanistic astrology, someone with too much 'earth' in their chart might seek a person with 'fire' qualities of intuition, creativity, vitality and adventure.[23] The chosen individual, who carries what we most fear or desire, becomes essential to our wholeness. To be complete we need to possess her. That obsessive feeling of wanting to eat the beloved alive is perhaps partly fuelled by the yearning to be whole.

The irony of projection is that while the lover experiences all the focus and meaning of her life as being with the beloved, in fact the beloved is an (often unwitting) actor in the lover's own internal drama. The beloved is chosen for the behaviour and feelings she catalyses in the lover, the qualities she draws to the surface, the buttons she happens to push. What is so magical about the person is that s/he illuminates the *lover's* internal landscape. As Raymond Durgnat writes of the role Jeanne Moreau plays in the film *Les Amants*: 'although she is seduced, in the sense that he lures her to follow him through the magical landscape, the landscape is herself, her own desires. His role is little more than that of a *porteur* in a romantic ballet.'[24] The power, the joy, is actually our own, but we rarely feel it as such. We need another to find ourselves, while we think we are finding them.

Ultimately, this can appear a rather sordid view of falling in love: we limp along appropriating others to fill gaps in ourselves, we latch on to them like vampires. Our own vitality and power in creating the situation remain unrecognised. Is it peculiar to patriarchy and capitalism that people have such large gaps that need filling? As people with more psychic scars, more unused potential, fewer outlets for self-realisation, are women in our society perhaps particularly prone to construct fantasies and seek completeness in another through these means?

However, we can also recognise that projection is a way of growing. It is possible to re-own, to reclaim what you are hooked on to the other person for. This process can be carried out quite explicitly in the therapy relationship, where the patient is sometimes encouraged to transfer feelings (which may be quite passionate) on to the therapist. In this case, as Perls points out:

> The therapist is supposed to have all the properties which are missing in this person. So, first the therapist provides the person with the opportunity to discover what he [she] needs – the missing parts that he [she] has alienated and given up to the world. Then the therapist must provide the opportunity, the situation in which the person can grow. And the means is that we frustrate the patient in such a way that he [she] is forced to develop his [her] own potential (my parentheses).[25]

Even in a personal love relationship, it is possible to recognise those magnetic, coveted qualities as one's own, and to work to express them more oneself.

Perhaps one way of understanding falling out of love is that the projection, which is often inaccurate, suddenly falls through. When the images which have been projected on to the beloved shatter, the person feels betrayed, 'as if "part of myself" had been taken away; and it has, but only because that part of myself, that image of self, was given to the other in the first place.'[26] Using another person as a symbol of our own potential can probably never stand the test of exposure to real life and actual contact for a great length of time. When the power given to a symbol is reclaimed, or recognised as inappropriate, the scales fall and we are left with just an ordinary-seeming person again.

In the meantime, however, the individual in love may have undergone enormous psychological and physical changes: the impact of such a powerful process of projection allows a suspension of normal beliefs, tensions and behaviour patterns, making space for new patterns to form. In the Seth books about the nature of human consciousness, Jane Roberts suggests that major problems can be shifted by any form of 'conversion':

> Under that general term I include strong emotional arousal and fresh emotional involvement, affiliation, or sense of belonging. This may involve religion, politics, art, or simply falling in love.
>
> In all of these areas the problem, whatever its nature or cause, is . . . 'magically' transferred to another facet of activity, projected away from the self. Huge energy blocks are moved . . .
>
> Love, as it is often experienced, allows an individual to take his [her] sense of self-worth from another for a time, and to at least momentarily let the other's belief in his [her] goodness supersede his [her] own beliefs in lack of worth. Again, I make a distinction between this and a greater love in which two individuals, knowing their own worth, are able to give and to receive.[27]

The upheaval associated with falling in love may, then, be a signal or catalyst of major personal change. In societies which offer more structures to mark such changes (whether through politics, art, religion, rituals or rites of passage), we may wonder whether falling in love looms as large as in our own. A key element in the process seems to be the ability temporarily to transcend personal limitations and boundaries. The psychosynthesis school of therapy suggests that an external ideal or figure can be a link to the higher Self which is reflected and symbolised in that figure.[28] You lose yourself temporarily in that figure in order to re-form. The psychological shake-up opens the way to a regrouping of the personality in a more coherent and unified form. In traditional language, the person 'drowns', 'dissolves', or is 'consumed' by the 'fires' of passion: again we find the implication of love as an agent of transformation.

Another angle on understanding falling in love has been to compare it to the overwhelming experience of childhood love for the mother, and to see it as some kind of regression to that early situation. This link is at the core of much traditional language about love, from the endearment 'baby', to the descriptive language about the loss of identity, the melting or dissolving, the all-consuming wanting, the return to an irrational or pre-rational state, the deep yearning and nostalgia as if for something which has been irrevocably lost. A woman in love can feel as totally vulnerable, as deeply intimate, as passionately identified with another, as a newborn baby with her mother. Perhaps it is some unanswered need for that time, or the premature loss of that childlike aspect of ourselves as we learnt the adult female role of caring, coping and servicing, which leaves a part of our being still crying out with open mouth for mother-love, and desperate to recreate it. As Melanie Klein puts it: 'However gratifying it is in later life to express thoughts and feelings to a congenial person, there remains an unsatisfied longing for an understanding without words – ultimately for the earliest relation with the mother.'[29]

If this need is part of the power behind falling in love, it might explain why intimacy and skin contact are sometimes more central to it than the act of sex itself. The yearning is perhaps not so much for orgasm as for symbiosis. This view would explain why the joy of falling in love is often very close to pain. Given the conditions of mothering in our society, few of us had a completely satisfactory early relationship with our mother, or were able to grow away from it in our own time. Recreating the same deep bond, it is hard for us to believe that the closeness will not turn sour or be withdrawn as happened with our original mother; perhaps we even unconsciously choose people who will fail us in exactly the same way that our mother did. This may be why the pain seems in some way precious. Perhaps we continually recreate the same scenario, hoping always that we can in this way free ourselves from it, that we can make a new ending.

Jane Rule argues that a relationship based on dependent mother–love is degrading and doomed to failure. She comments:

> I am always nervous about the suggestion that, as lesbians, we should mother each other, though I understand that the image comes from our first source of love. Our mothers are also the first source of rejecting power against whom we screamed our dependent rage. As adults, if we cry out for that mother–love, the dependent rage inevitably follows, and what is even more disconcerting is that, given total attention and sympathy, we are soon restless to be free, for we aren't any longer children.[30]

In this gripping re-run of our early emotional lives, it seems that men can stand in for our mummies, or women represent our daddies. What is riveting is the *internal* dynamic, the replay of the tragic drama. As Miriam tells Jackson in *Small Changes*:

> I wasn't a loved child, and I have those mechanisms of the woman who gets hooked on trying to make someone love her. You become the father I was never pretty enough to please. You become the mother who never found my best good enough.[31]

In her book, *Room to Breathe*, Jenny James states that for her the endless re-enactment is of winning not her mother's, but her father's love. She describes how, in one relationship after another, an inaccessible and desired person becomes unwanted as soon as they are won over and thus cease to recreate the right degree of childhood pain.[32]

But what is it that makes certain people 'right' to stand in for our mothers and fathers in this way? Is it, as some believe, the recognition of a twin soul reincarnated from the passion of a past life?[33] Or is that they are in the right place at the right time and imagination does the rest? There may be superficial parallels in personality and behaviour, but sometimes more invisible connections seem to be at work.

Here it seems relevant to examine how falling in love is experienced in the body. It is often associated with acute physical sensations, such as stomach churning, warm glows, tingles down the spine, and so on. However, these sensations are rarely investigated or correlated to our emotional experience.[34] Our ignorance of the body is so immense that I can only mention certain aspects of our experience which need to be discussed and understood at much greater depth.

Though I have said the experience may not be primarily a sexual one, it is certainly physical. We are to a certain extent aware of how the five senses are involved. Eyes are often the magnet for attraction, as in 'love at first sight'. The voice of the beloved is often important: in fairy stories a person may fall in love with the sound of another's singing. Taste and smell are perhaps more important than we consciously recognise. Techniques apparently now exist for odour 'fingerprinting' of human bodies: perhaps some people carry a smell which reaches us very effectively or echoes the irresistible smell of mother. The implication of recognising the role of sight, hearing and smell may be that we can be physically sensitive to a person before there is any contact. Our bodies may respond to a stranger in far more ways than we are consciously aware of. Touch is also important. Here a woman recounts a common experience: 'When I first met J., I was sitting next to her in a chair. My hand accidentally brushed against hers and I felt a charge between us like electricity, as if there was a current between our two hands.'[35]

Here we have to stop and reconsider. Another vocabulary is entering the accounts. Why is it that one person's touch, given it is equally smooth or gentle or hot or cold, feels so different from another's and can galvanise us, or not? Why is it that one person's eyes say 'Hello', while another's reach into the soul and draw it magnetically? Here we are moving beyond the generally recognised powers of the five senses. What do we believe the eyes do when they 'mesmerise'?

What do the eyes and voice do when they 'hypnotise'? The language of Alison Buckley's poem is illuminating:

> In the first splash of meeting, first half-second
> I looked; I saw she was open like a radar-scanner
> picking up every prickly tingle from me. Smiles zoomed
>     out
> undulating quanta of warmth, racing each other
> penetrating, and bursting inside my eyes
> travelling light years inside my head.

Radar, electricity. A contact which zooms, races, penetrates, undulates like radio waves. This is precisely the kind of language used by esoteric anatomy to describe the phenomenon of the 'energy body' which is thought to interpenetrate and surround our physical body.

The theory is that each person has an energy-field similar to, but not identical with, an electromagnetic energy-field.[36] This 'electro-magnetic' energy runs through the body along channels and radiates outwards from it. An inner layer of radiation close to the skin surface has been recorded photographically by Kirlian aura photography[37] which shows variations in the aura depending on the health, temper and state of mind of the person. The theory also suggests that people's energy-fields interact with each other. We can respond unconsciously to the energy emitted by another, and may be attracted or repelled by conflicts or resonances in the energy-fields.

This theory has some resonances in our everyday experience. There is the language of 'good vibes' and 'bad vibes' and of being 'drawn' to or getting a 'buzz' from someone. There are the metaphors of electricity from the accounts I have quoted, and many people will recognise the experience of feeling 'drained' by spending time with a depressed person. Some people may have experienced the movement of 'energy' in their body during yoga exercises, or may have met it as 'body energy' in bioenergetic massage or therapy; others may relate it to the 'meridians' of acupuncture.

This language could be used to give expression to the powerful rushes of feeling between lovers. One way of describing falling in love could be as a bonding between two people who have a particularly acute and needed exchange of energy to make with one another. This might explain the intense feelings of separation and difference combined with feelings of kinship: like two pieces of a jigsaw puzzle, each has what the other needs to make her whole. This 'fine' energy contact has been described as a sixth sense which imbues and informs the contact made through the other five. It sums up the feeling of wordless connection as a movement of energy between two people. It could account for the sense of under-cutting normal ways of relating, as well as the sense of being physically potentiated, experiencing intimacy and close contact, without sex necessarily being the prime mover.

I am suggesting this approach as another of the theoretical frameworks which we could use for understanding the process of falling in love. It is not a popular approach, but it interests me personally as it provides a language for certain aspects of the experience which other theories ignore. We do not have to 'believe' in it, any more than we have to 'believe' in projection, but we can explore the usefulness of each framework. Nor do I see any of the theories described in this (personal and certainly incomplete) survey as incompatible or mutually exclusive alternatives. To say that two people have mutually interlocking energy-fields may be another way of saying that one has been building up tension which the other can release; or that one smells like the other's mother; or that they are formed so that it is easy for each to project on to the other; or that they fill holes in each other's personality. The same process can be understood on a number of different levels. To talk about 'energy' does not exclude looking at things in psychological and social terms, although we need to develop a more subtle framework to combine these understandings.

As an ineffable, intense and other-wordly experience, being in love has been compared to religious ecstasy. It has also been suggested that sexual relationships more often have spiritual overtones for women than for men. Béla Grunberger writes: 'As man's sexual life is focused on immediate instinctual relief, woman's love is also located in time, but she dreams of eternity.'[38] Socially we can explain this male/female difference, if it exists, as a result of our upbringing and conditioning around sexually and relationships; but what is being referred to may be the greater facility women experience in tuning in to fine energy. Alexander Lowen defines the soul as 'the sense or feeling in a person of being part of a larger or universal order',[39] and sees it as the result of our body energy interacting with the energy around us in the world and in the universe, which gives the feeling of being part of something bigger than yourself. Perhaps the strong link which occurs when we fall in love can open us up to these wider connections. Perhaps it is an experience which opens the 'lines' between ourselves and the world.[40] In a culture which denies spirituality outside the confines of established religion, falling in love may have become unusually important as one of our few routes to an experience of the transcendent. It has been understood as a distortion of a deep urge to love the world which through social pressures gets funnelled into one person.

In this, falling in love typifies the contradictory nature of our experiences under capitalism and patriarchy, our efforts to be human in a world organised along inhuman lines. The positive is so entwined with the negative. Falling in love makes us feel strong, but it also makes us feel weak. It is liberating, but it is also obsessive. It tunes us in to our love and warmth, but also to our gaping need and vulnerability. It reaches out, yet it is highly individualistic. Even the much-vaunted melting and closeness has been open to challenge. Though spiritual disciplines may suggest that 'Love is the recognition of the same consciousness in another as in oneself ',[41] others assert that true contact involves a recognition of separateness and differences.[42] From the perspective of political activity, falling in love has been seen as regressive, self-indulgent, privatised, time-wasting.

So how should we deal with it from a perspective of feminism? Should we struggle against these tendencies and feelings in ourselves as counter-productive? I don't think so. Rather, I feel we should take that power and vitality and work with them. If we were not damaged and empty, if our life-experiences had been different, perhaps our loving would not be shot through with need, pain and obsession. But we are as we are, and we have to start from there. Rather than denigrating falling in love, we could see it as a healthy response to a crazy world and perhaps one of the stratagems our organism uses to survive. Perhaps it gives a release where a release is badly needed. On many levels it seems to be a vehicle for the expression of the suppressed. We could see it as a distorted expression of real needs, but in some ways it may be a healthy choice for us: a lifeline enabling us to give and receive love in a way we usually cannot. The idea of love may have been misused, but to deny that we want and need intimacy with others is to avoid the whole issue.[43] We probably need both symbiosis with and separateness from other people, and what is important is for us to develop access to both, to open the channels so that we can move easily into each as we need, instead of lurching in juddering spasms from one to the other, out of control.[44] Instead of attempting to censor or dismiss these passionate feelings, we could work creatively with them. Perhaps the question is not why we have these 'incorrect' and humiliating experiences and how we can stop having them, but rather why that intensity and vitality of contact is confined to such a localised area; and how we can gain more access to experiencing and directing that vitality in other areas of our lives.

How can we do this? The first and crucial step seems to be owning our own power in the situation. We use the term 'falling' in love which disguises the fact that we have chosen to leap and have abdicated responsibility for our experience. The feelings, fantasies and sensations that possess us are in fact our own. We say that another 'makes' us feel unbelievable excitement, but actually the excitement is ours.[45] If we can feel it in one situation, we can feel it in another. We need to cease thinking of others as the source of reference point for our feelings, and recognise our own role more clearly.

One way of doing this is to become more conscious of the stages and details of the process of falling in love. It is time to stop muddying our experience by talking about things which 'mysteriously happened' to us. What exactly *did* happen? Where did I feel it in my body? When have I experienced similar sensations? Who or what triggered it? What did they do? What did I do? What happens if I do something different? Gradually we can learn the paths into all these experiences for ourselves.[46] One area to clarify is the link for each of us with sexuality. What turns us on sexually? What makes us fall in love? What is the difference? We need to get more familiar with the body's language. As Jane Rule comments:

> Sex is not so much an identity as a language which we have for so long been forbidden to speak that most of us learn only the crudest of its vocabulary and grammar. If we are to get past the pattern of dominance and submission, of possessive greed, we must outgrow love as fever, as 'the tragic necessity of human life', and speak in tongues that set us free to be loving equals.[47]

Body awareness seems crucial. How can we retain a sense of our own power when we are draining out of our bodies to identify with another? One woman reports realising that 'the most important thing was not to make him love me but for me to love aliveness.'[48] Our experience of aliveness is in and through our body's sensations and processes: this is our ground, our sustenance, our inner richness, and we lose our power if we abandon it.

There are other aspects of the process with which we can get more familiar. What if I start a relationship with a slow burner rather than a flash in the pan? What do I gain or lose? If falling in love is a reaction to suppression, what exactly do I need to release: anger? sexual desire? grief? political energy? What other ways do I have of breaking out, of expressing what is held in? If projection is involved, we can ask: What *are* my 'fancies' about this person I fancy? When have I had similar fantasies? How do they connect to fantasies I have about myself? What does this person have that I need or believe that I lack? How can I bring those qualities into my life independently of them?[49] What does this person potentiate in me, and how could I potentiate it in myself? We might ask: Is this person like my mother/father? In what ways does s/he love or fail me like my mother/father did? Do I want to change that and make a new ending?

If falling in love makes us feel spiritual, what else has the same effect? If we feel something similar when massaging or meditating or gardening or listening to music, we can watch those experiences. What are the situations, the ingredients, the states of mind that predispose us to feel that way? Thus we can learn how to choose certain experiences and not others. Falling in love is not unfathomable: the fathoms are ours, and we can learn to swim in our own depths without diminishing their power and beauty.

Another step we can take is consciously to broaden the scope of our loving feelings. Part of this may be to realise that we 'fall in love' in situations far from the socially recognised romantic or sexual ones. Because our culture does not validate such feelings, we tend to dismiss them ourselves. In accordance with prevailing economic and social pressures, we envision a hierarchy of relationships with the perfect couple at the top, while 'chance encounters with . . . children, old people, gas fitters, kite-flyers, just don't have a look in.'[50] Here a woman describes a situation which would never normally be graced with the title of 'being in love':

'Oh Johnny, it's you!' When my granny was dying, my brother looked after her and they developed a love relationship. When he visited her in hospital after an operation, she greeted him as she would a lover. There was an intimacy and excitement and interest and tenderness between them which looked to me like two people who are in love.[51]

We hear of non-sexual relationships between women which carry passion, fascination, delight and a peculiar resonance for the two friends involved. Mothers describe being 'in love' with their babies, intimately bonded by a magic line as strong as an umbilical cord. And it does not stop with people. A teenager may claim to be 'in love' with a horse. And what about moments of work which we can suddenly connect to, or the love-affair with a particular career or activity which may last stormily over many years? Or the times when ideas seize us and obsess us? Or the feeling of uplift on a mass demonstration when we feel intensely towards every other human being there? We can't 'fall in love' with ourselves, or with a country, or with a movement. Perhaps recognising and nurturing those experiences can be one way of diffusing the passionate intimacy and contact of 'falling in love' into wider areas of our lives. Enormous power and vitality is involved: imagine what we could do with it. As *Ink* pointed out:

> Puritans should note what while . . . resistance can take the form of the worker's absolute need for food and shelter, it is also manifested in the desire for excitement instead of boredom, love instead of politeness. The desire for love, conscious of itself and what opposes it, would become a determination to transform the whole of human behaviour and its economic roots.[52]

I would like to believe that it could. The first step may be to accept and know our own experience better, and to move outwards from there. We may be able to make the first step towards the transforming our love from a bewildering passion for one person to a deep-rooted lust for all of life. We can at least try.

From *Sex and Love: New Thoughts on Old Contradictions*, edited by Sue Cartledge and Joanna Ryan, published by The Women's Press.

# SALLY CLINE
## Convent Girls and Impossible Passions

Today women, who have always know about passion, are searching for new kinds. They believe they will find them in or through celibacy. Women talk about the 'freedom' to discover a passion that is not lust. How absurd that we should need such a freedom, that the current obsession with genital activity should make us feel that we have lost it. For women have always found pleasure in a multitude of magnificent passions. Women can be passionate about their homes, their children, their families, their extended families, whom they protect and defend fiercely and with great love. Some women are passionate about roses; others about art. Some feel a passion for God; others for meditation.

Women cannot afford to pigeon-hole their passions; they have to let them slide over the edges of their busy lives, fitting them in when there is time (and usually there is not). Perhaps celibacy is one way of offering women time for old passions, space to discover new ones.

I dare say my own passions will seem quirky to some, but to me they are compelling. They nourish my daily routine, whether or not it includes sex. I have noticed that when I am celibate my passions assume a greater significance. I am passionate about books: poetry, biography, philosophy, any time. Fiction 'for daytime train journeys. Crime for nights. I never leave the house without a book to read tucked into my bag. I am most passionate about the writings of Virginia Woolf. Her framed photo has been hung above every desk I have written at.

I have a passion for travel. It prevents brooding. It unleashes my imagination. Watching the waves break on the shore minimizes my own disorders. So does waiting for the dawn to break. Or there is the passion of walking in

Cornwall, framed by the mountains, watching the bright turquoise of the sea turn to sombre navy with grey lines and swirls, wondering if the famous Sennen fog will soon surround me.

A passion for words. The rush and urgency to find just the right word. Will that word or this word light up a room, brush over a character? Will the words knit together, will they spirit me away?

A passion for silence and solitude. The relief of being with someone who understands without words, who goes away for long periods, and leaves me alone with my books and my pottering. The blissful knowledge that I have several days at a time, up in an attic, away from the racket of life, which no one is scheduled to interrupt or disturb. In solitude I can hang the walls of my mind with bright coloured canvas. I can be who I am beneath the skin.

By contrast the passion of good conversation; intimate friendship; the feeling of loving and being loved by friends, by family; motherhood. That extraordinary surge of sensation when I watched my (then) baby daughter swim her first few strokes in an adult swimming pool. Did I really have something to do with creating her? More than twenty years later, participating in her excitement when she purchased and moved into her first house. Over the years, sharing suppers on a tray in front of the television, with Vic, the youngest of the girls I helped bring up, both of us snuggled in on the sofa beside Fruitcake and Bod, the two black cats.

A passion for politics. The warm feeling of being with those who share the values I hold precious. Marching with other women for peace, or against male violence, or for abortion rights or to honour gay pride. In later years, working and walking in the rain at Greenham, feeling part of something that absolutely has to change the world or we are doomed. Lighting candles, braving the storms, clutching the railings, glaring at the men on the other side. Passion and politics, strength and support, everywhere one looked.

A passion for dancing. I remember as a child in the forties, my mother and my Aunt Het teaching me to do the Charleston by holding on to the back of a chair. Then the three of us dancing it together at big Jewish weddings and barmitzvahs. Today, taking a sudden decision to join a jazz dance class. Wondering if I am too old, wondering if I should have bought a leotard. Then the fever of dancing takes over, and the music that pumps out the world's energy restores mine.

Colours. I have a passion for certain colours. The flare of brown and orange autumn leaves crackling beneath my feet, crisp in white lace-up shoes. Brown and orange taking me back in time to the flaming brown and orange sitting room in which I spent my most intense years. Memory ensures I shall always have a passion for brown and orange.

An old passion for food and a new passion for gardening. Planting sweet-smelling night stock near the back kitchen, and a mass of lavender bushes by the front door. If I leave the doors open on a summer's day, there are amazing smells everywhere as I wander through the house. The excitement of picking new potatoes I had actually grown, matching them to garden radishes, leeks and spring onions, adding Indian spices, creating another meal without going to the local shops. How proud I felt.

A passion for certain pieces of music. Verdi's *Rigoletto*, my father's favourite opera. 'Sharm El Sheikh', a piece for mouth organ and orchestra, composed for the Israeli troops fighting in the place of that name during the Six-Day War. In the sixties, the memorable experience of holding my small daughter's hand, as I watched her musician father play that music for those troops.

Pop music of 1978, the year I fell in love. Joan Armatrading. The LP bought the same year. That first weekend. We were so wrapped up in conversation – what was it we were talking about? – we let candle grease drip on to the record.

The passion invoked by a sensual celibate relationship, conducted for geographical reasons, largely by post and telephone. Rushing to the door as the post arrives. Ripping open the envelopes that never have postcodes. Don't you know that without postcodes, heady tales of adventure take three times as long to reach the recipient? Waiting in, high with excitement, on the nights scheduled for phone calls. The joy of lending each other books by post, trying to read each other's minds. Spending a fortune on postage stamps.

We have no adequate framework for the feelings engendered by these sensual celibate relationships explored by women in the late twentieth century – perhaps in some ways they mirror romantic friendships of the nineteenth century – but what is not in doubt is the passion that is attached to them.

Finally, beyond or beneath these passions lurks another, new and growing. Possibly it is emerging snail-like through years of slow change and consistent challenge. Like many of the women I talked to, I feel that I have started on a path towards something beyond my imaginings. It is something that is not quite there, that requires constant attention, demands increasing awareness, may well be enhanced by celibacy and solitude.

Passions are as personal as fingerprints. These are some of mine. Your list will be different. Women are exploring them through celibacy. Many women are quite simply passionate about celibacy itself.

Is a passion for celibacy an impossible possibility? The genital myth would contend that it is.

I raise the question because, in our sexually saturated society, the juxtaposition of those two nouns, passion and celibacy, has an incompatible sound. For in our culture the term 'passion' has largely been reserved for sexual activity, or as one woman put it, for 'great sexual love', a good example of the romantic ideology at work.

Although Polly Blue was one woman who, through living a new life infused with positive celibate energy, had arrived at a radically different and wider understanding of the meaning of passion – for her, celibacy had opened up possibilities that were a mixture of personal, political, spiritual and sexual passions – for many women, not being 'allowed' to view passion as appropriate in a celibate situation is the first obstacle they have to confront when deciding to become celibate.

I myself have had a certain struggle with the notion, which is due in part to my legacy as a Jewish girl who was educated for a brief period at a Catholic convent. This seemed to be an educational rather than a religious habit in my family, for two of my girl cousins were also sent to convent schools for substantial periods of their childhood.

As convent girls we were taught early the challenge and fascination of the convergence of impossible possibilities. The Catholic faith taught us that bodies were irrelevant, that it was the life of the spirit which counted, yet the nuns talked incessantly about bodies, about mortification of the flesh, about temptations that could only be fleshy, material, and all too human. To attain the higher potential of the spiritual self one learnt to subdue what one cheeky convent girl in an older class called 'impossible longings'. Being a girl who let her longings get the better of her, she did something in those days classed as unspeakable. In a free period when she should have been writing up her lessons, or reflecting on the proofs of the existence of Our Lord, or praying for a schoolfriend who was going through a crisis of faith, she wrote a letter to a boy, telling him in lurid detail exactly what she wanted. Inevitably she was found out, every rude word of the letter was perused by the shocked sisters, and we saw her no more. I say we 'saw her no more' because I have no idea if she was expelled, exchanged with a student from another school who did not have 'longings', or whisked away to another place on a flapping black habit. At the time, her vanishment (or banishment) seemed entirely mysterious, but I was left with the firm impression that there went a girl who would never attain the State of Grace, a girl who had failed to achieve the highest possibility. Being a young girl who had 'longings' of a certain kind myself, I became worried, but I knew without any doubt that temporarily I should have to subdue them, for I did not want to end up like her.

Another impossible possibility that faced us in those convent years, was the one about heaven. We learnt at a very young age that the possibility of going to heaven was an offer for all 'good' (ie chaste and compliant) convent girls, even

Jewish ones, but we also learnt that there was no easy access. Struggle, a key word in our Jewish home, was also a key word in the Catholic faith. The way upward to heaven was fraught with obstacles, and riddled with restrictive rules which even the best of us, which I was not, invariably broke.

Irish writer Clare Boylan, who thought of her convent school background as a symbol of 'aspiration to the unattainable' recalls the difficulties of achieving entrance to heaven which is never the less regarded as a genuine possibility. She describes it as 'a universal symbol for expectation and ambition, that I think anybody with a Jewish background would probably understand.'[1]

She is of course absolutely right. Being Jewish informs a woman's consciousness for all time. However, so does being a convent girl, no matter how transiently. A literary penchant for confession was one inheritance I received from the Catholic faith, as transmitted by the nuns. An early association of intense sex with intense sin was another. I suspect my interest in goals and rewards developed from the fact that the convent would offer us encouragement and awards of blue ribbons and shiny medals for special spiritual achievement. Excessive modesty of both body and spirit was something I recall being demanded of me, but to my mortification I did not win any blue ribbons on either count.

I did however learn to slap down in myself any lurking suspicions of superiority. As humility and obedience (as well as chastity of course) were the three big moral qualities, 'acting superior' invited strict penances. Being a child who feared and eluded confrontation and punishment, I did not easily court penance, and would attempt instead to charm or bluff, with a new batch of manipulatively good behaviour, one of the less severe (and less clear-sighted) sisters. It was only later that I realised the irony of a situation where these strong, independent, tough women, who led autonomous and seemingly fulfilled lives, endlessly taught us the passive and stereotypically feminine qualities of humility and obedience. The nuns were hardly conforming housewives and mothers; they had broken the mould, why did they not expect us to?

During my time as a pupil in this North London convent, this relevant and pertinent question simply never occurred to me. Instead I would puzzle over spiritual matters I did not fully understand, as I watched the nuns marching in a long procession through the assembly hall. There was the smell of incense as they walked, and a clickety noise of the rosary beads slightly swaying. The nuns talked constantly of the virtue and suffering of the virgin saints, who became heroines to most of us. We knew that to emulate our idols we too must subdue something the sisters called 'fleshy appetites'. I remember picturing sex as a huge, squashy, red tomato!

Oh yes, we all got a clear vision very early on, about what celibacy was *not*. But what was it? Was it the same as chastity? We heard a great deal about chastity. We all knew the stories of our heroines, the amazing Teresa of Avila, and the bitterly sad Bernadette of Lourdes, both of whom had undeniably been chaste, and had undeniably suffered. Saint Teresa had been paralysed, and Saint Bernadette had died of tuberculosis and, according to the nuns, they never complained. Could we feel the same passion for the chaste state as the nuns and the saints felt? Should we have to suffer for it first? Suffering was very high up on my convent agenda, just as it was integral to the Jewish way of life. You do not emerge from the Diaspora without heavy suffering, as my uncles and grandparents bore witness. It was hardly surprising that inhabiting as I did these two redolently ritualistic worlds (one smelling of garlic and chopped liver, the other of fresh flowers and incense, both focused on pain and patience, agony and ecstasy), I soon began to believe that suffering was significant in itself. I think this view had something to do with my positive adoption, as a teenager, of existential philosophy with its necessary component of angst.

I remember once wondering whether it was celibacy the nuns had tacked on with severe stitches to their austere black habits. There was certainly some indefinable aura that attached to their skirts and their presence, a dignity, a centred control, a movement of love and spiritual strength, both outwards towards us and inwards towards themselves and Our Lady, that was entirely different from the atmosphere engendered by my talkative, worldly, affectionate, bickering, Jewish family, who spoke Yiddish when they wanted to discuss matters 'unsuitable for the children's ears', which gave me a similar feeling of displacement and alienation to the one I felt when I heard Mass spoken in Latin.

At home, my father and uncles were interested in me and in my progress, but they were more interested in their business schemes, their law briefs, their tailoring schedules, and in the strange, secretive and enclosed world of the Freemasons, whose masculine materialistic rituals clashed even more strongly with the feminine and spiritual rituals of the convent, than did even my Jewish heritage. My mother and my aunties, whose own interests generally revolved around the men, food for the men, food for the rest of the family, and stories of the most successful offspring, wanted me to succeed and of course to keep all the rules. They hardly noticed that during my time at the convent (an episode which centred on educational success and geographical moves) I was faced with two entirely different and often competing sets of rules.

The nuns on the other hand noticed everything. Because they did not have men and meals to cater for, their devotion to duty, and to us, the young charges who formed a large part of their duty, was tireless and total. I felt they were interested in everything I did, and far too interested in the things I did wrong, which is how I learnt so much, so swiftly, about confession.

Today, having talked to a great many nuns, I understand that one of the greatest gifts the nuns gave to us, their girls, the gift of passionate attention, came from their celibate philosophy that 'loves all' and 'loves all well'. Their belief that not focusing on one special person made better sense of their celibate lives, allowed them to regard each of us with what seemed to a child's eyes like a very special concentration. Many years later as an adult, I had a similar feeling when I was discussing celibacy with nuns in a Canadian theological college. In theory, I was there to interview them; in practice it was I who was put gracefully and attentively under the white light.

Novelist Jean Rhys, who at the age of fourteen went happily as a boarder to a convent, at a later age than I did, remembers the nuns teaching order and chastity, that 'most precious possession', that 'flawless crystal that once broken can never be mended'.[2] The celibate state to young girls in convents was the state of preciousness and safety in stern contrast to sexual activity which in those days represented danger or the devil's work. I clearly recall sex as peril but I do not remember it standing for passion, because all of us knew that what the nuns were passionate about was Jesus Christ. All of us knew that he was to be the receptacle of our love also. His arms, spread over the cross, invited us to offer up our fervent, youthful, girlish passions. As Germaine Greer wrote in an essay about her Catholic childhood, Christ 'really is the archetypal lover', and convent educated girls (of whatever religion), prostrate and pining on church floors, have little trouble believing it.[3]

You do not have to be a Catholic to bear the imprint of convent life. I still think visions and voices should be taken seriously; I still believe that organisation and structure is the way to contain a wanton wildness, I still find compelling in women the combination of fierce strength and unremitting modesty, which the sisters so ardently illustrated. I still find scruples endlessly absorbing. It is no coincidence that having been reared as a child on scruples and moral problems I should have elected ethics as the major paper of my philosophy degree. A favourite scruple, which I spent a long time pondering during my childhood, was what could a girl do or not do in the way of French kissing or masturbation if she wanted to avoid committing a mortal sin? Chastity, as I recall, was always part of my bargaining power with either Jesus or Our Lady. I would suggest something along the lines that if I was allowed just a trifling amount of French kissing, hardly putting my tongue inside the boy's mouth, then in return I would offer five more years' chastity. Generally Jesus and Our Lady did not deign to reply.

I grew up with a staunch and tiresome devotion to duty, instilled as much by the nuns who taught me briefly as by my Jewish family, whose teaching still lurks (sometimes uncomfortably) inside my head.

Novelist Jean Rhys recalled from her convent days the nuns' advice that to go and work very hard at something was the best way to drive out the devil.[4] My own convent inheritance in the matter of the struggle against the devil's machinations (a struggle I have frequently lost) has been this belief in hard work and duty, and a knowledge that part of my duty was to pay passionate attention to those I cared for, in the way that the nuns paid passionate attention to us, the girls they loved.

At some level I understood very early that a non-sexually active love can be just as passionate and just as absorbing as a genitally rooted one; and that such a love has at its centre the idea of being fully focused or intentional. But when I was an adolescent, many years after leaving the convent, enthralled in the first flush of unconsummated lust for the marvellous and miraculous Michael Flower (a boy much older than myself who paid me almost no attention and broke my fragile sixth former's heart), I had no way of differentiating or weighing up these two kinds of passion. As young heady girls out in the world are wont to do, I simply threw away the non-genital passion, and for several years, co-opted by the prevailing culture of my time, concentrated on the genital excitement of sex with lamentable indiscrimination, and a feverish enthusiasm that might have been better applied to my studies.

In the sixth form I developed a desire to be a saint which hotly conflicted with the guilty knowledge that for a girl like me, sin was always just around the corner. Even after a considerable period at an ordinary state school, I still believed that spotty boys would go berserk with passion if they could see the shape of my bum through my navy gym knickers on the hockey field.

I was, as you see, a child in a muddle over passion and celibacy. In the early years passion represented on the one hand spiritual devotion to Christ, a deep and caring love for those who were important to us on earth, and, most significantly in terms of the subject of this study, the independence of the strong female spirit; yet on the other hand, there was the matter of lust which lurked outside the convent doors. The outside world called *that* 'passion', while the nuns, who never made that mistake, and sharply differentiated true passion from what they saw as either temptation or sinful behaviour, were never the less passionate about putting it down.

A convent, as all ex-convent girls know, is the Home of Rules, chief amongst which is 'No Looseness', a rule which led me early to suspect that once you were let loose into the world, sin would await you at every corner. As writer Maeve Binchy, another ex-convent girl, said: 'I thought the world was going to be full of lust, and it was just waiting. The main thing I would have to do was beat it off because that was what the Church was all about, beating it off until the time was right.'[5] For Maeve Binchy, the time would be right within Christian marriage but certainly not before that. For a young Jewish ex-convent girl the timing was equally important, and somewhat more complex.

A Jewish background intensified the problems of passion and celibacy, the confusions that arose from sifting sex from sin from sacred states. Passion, if it existed at all for young Jewish girls, and it patently was *not* a necessary condition for a good Jewish life, was inextricably linked to sexual obedience and the marital bond to a Jewish man. In my family, as in most Jewish households, as soon as a young woman mentioned a young man's name, the first question would be 'Is he Jewish?' This was not a light matter. *Gehinnom*, the Hebrew name for hell, is reserved for Gentiles, and for Jewish women who have sex with non-Jewish men. Marriage to a non-Jew would be so out of the question that *Gehinnom* itself could not hold such a fallen Jewish woman.

If the young woman's answer to the key question was 'Yes

he is Jewish', she would be told: 'So you'll make a good marriage – then, maybe, will come the passion . . .' At this point there would be a knowing sigh from a mother or an aunty. Jewish mothers and Jewish aunties know that Jewish men are encouraged to woo a woman sexually to a passionate state, so long as she is a legitimate Jewish wife. 'Win her over with words of graciousness and seductiveness. Hurry not to arouse her passion until her mood is ready, begin in love; let her "semination" (orgasm) take place first.'[6]

If the mother or the aunty did not have great hopes of the sexual skills of the young woman's betrothed she would wink and say pragmatically: 'So if there is no passion so then instead soon will be the babies.'

End of passion. End of discussion.

As for celibacy, my Jewish upbringing utterly contradicted my Catholic School, for unlike the latter where the self-chosen celibacy of the nuns was held in high esteem, where chastity and modesty were venerated above all else, in my Jewish home celibacy was seen as a substantially more impoverished condition than marriage. Of greater significance is the fact that celibacy only applied to men. Jewish women were not regarded as celibate; they were always seen as virginal, as waiting to get married, or to be married off. This idea that virginity is merely a physiological condition, a waiting state, that is different in essence from positive celibacy is one to which I shall return.

Thomas Szasz reminds us: 'The Christian teaching against marriage and for chastity (that is for marriage to Jesus) could be regarded as an act of liberation from compulsory Jewish matrimony . . . [so] the faithful Jew finds pleasure in marital coitus and procreation; the faithful Christian in celibate chastity.'[7]

In both my childhood religions it was men (either literally or in the shape of Christ in the early years, the Rabbis in the later years) who were prioritised and served with a passionate obedience. In the secular ideologies that stand as a context to marriage and family life it is still men who are prioritised. The idea that self-chosen celibacy might be a state of independence in which the female self is prioritised, that moreover celibacy might be part of a woman's sexuality, rather than opposed to it, and that women might attach to it with a passion, as much earthly as spiritual, comes as a revolutionary idea to many non-religious women. But to the practising nuns in Great Britain and North America to whom I talked about the relationship of celibacy to sexuality, and the nature of the 'passion' attached to it, it appeared to be quite an ordinary idea.

Like the 'joyful, sexual, wise, funny and loving nuns' whom Polly Blue had known and admired, and who had been eager to tell her that 'they have bodies and are sexual', many nuns I talked to made similar statements.[8]

Two of the nuns I met were working as nurses out in communities in Canada. Sister Anne who was forty-one told me:

> My male patients know I am a nun and have taken a vow of celibacy, but it doesn't stop them from asking me out. They obviously see me as sexual. I see myself as sexual too, but in a different way. Celibacy for me is a way of life whereby I am able to express my sexuality not in a non-sexual way but in a way that calls me to love well. Sometimes it seems hard to give up the idea of being loved by one person but I am immersed in the struggle to try and love all.
>
> I see celibacy as a sexual state because I am a sexual being expressing my love, sometimes a caregiver's love, sometimes a love for a friend or relative, in a celibate way. Touch and intimacy are part of my sexuality, which the Church used to think of as negative but does not any more.

Sister Mary, a few years younger than Sister Anne, doing a similar nursing job, confirmed the importance of touch:

> As a nun out in the community, I do hands-on healing in my work as a nurse. The way I heal, the way I touch people physically is a part of my sexual being. Sometimes people, well, men, expect a response from me, that I might feel but

I cannot give. Centring myself on God and touching others in relationships along the way are both parts of my celibate sexual self in service.

I asked Sister Charles, a nun who taught in another theological college, whether she saw herself as sexual.

Oh yes, I have no doubts that I am sexual. I do not engage in sexual intercourse, but the sexuality that I live is like a pulse that goes right through me. There is an erotic part of who I am that is lived out in deep relationships of love. It is lived out also in prayer. I think there is a strong connection between eroticism and prayer. It is a connection that scares us, that we desire, that we do not quite know what to do with. Sexuality and spirituality are both the core of what it means to be a human, and to be a woman. There was a time when I would have denied my sexuality, denied the connection between the erotic and the religious, but not now. I think many of us have denied it in the past and it has caused sterility in religious experience. We are nuns vowed to celibacy but we are also women whose sexuality is focused on our call and on the work we do.

Some nuns to whom I talked have had a more overt struggle with the problem of the blurred lines between what it means to be sexual and what it means to be celibate. Sister Angela, who at fifty-three still lives in the community where she took her first vows, explained the contradictions and conflicts of being a 'sexually celibate' nun.

When I first entered the community, we were not encouraged to give voice to any sexual feelings we experienced. Particular friendships with other nuns were discouraged, and any closeness you might have felt towards other sisters was limited by what we all believed was appropriate behaviour for vowed nuns. I did not doubt that I was a sexual woman or that I had strong physical and emotional feelings for one or two others, but for many years there were no possibilities for anything like what you would call 'a relationship'. There were merely sexual undertones.

Ten years ago the times had changed sufficiently for issues of sexuality to be raised and discussed within the community. I had become very attached to another nun. I shall call her 'Marie'. We were reaching towards each other, she perhaps because she was many years younger than me, in a more explicit sexual way. I had to face what was happening and I had to think about my celibate vocation, my vow of chastity, in the light of my feelings for my particular friend, and of hers for me.

She had been brave enough to voice them. I had finally found the courage to respond. We had begun to spend more time than was appropriate together. We touched each other, we began to focus on each other. That was the worst (although at the time it seemed the best); that focus on each other. She wanted to express her love for me in a genitally intimate way but, like me, she also wanted to stay inside the community. It was a time of agony and indecision. She began to talk about wanting to spend years alone with me. She used new words like 'home' and 'together' that did not fit our circumstances as vowed nuns. Suddenly everything I had given my life for all these years seemed in jeopardy.

Sister Angela told me that she had loved Sister Marie and had been prepared to acknowledge that love, but her profound dilemma was that she was vowed to God.

I was vowed to love all. I knew that what she and I could have if we left the community might be intense or joyous, but I felt it would be too narrow, in some way more restricted than the love and bonding of a shared celibacy that remains pure. We talked and we talked. We finally decided that we had no choice, or that I had no choice.

We stayed in the community together for three years, experiencing the bonds of love but limiting their expression to only those ways which were compatible with our vocation. We talked about it to our superior who was gentle and understanding. From her I felt given the strength I needed to continue in this way. Unfortunately Marie my friend grew restless, and more depressed. Our love, which she felt had been contained, no longer uplifted her. Eventually in deep misery she left the community. I needed all the strength our love and bonding had given me to continue to ask for grace and to commit myself to God and all my sisters.

Sister Angela told me that she still loved Sister Marie, that she still thinks about her, but that she is still committed to the life of the community.

It would be facile to say that I feel better for having undergone that suffering. I don't feel better, I don't. How many times have I wished it had not brought such suffering? But my vow of celibacy means more to me now than before it had been tested. During the anxious sexually intimate times with her I felt possessed, I did not feel free to do my work for God. Sometimes now I am sad, but I am not focused on a single person. I feel I can act out my ministry in a more creative manner. My celibacy is pulsing with human emotion and spirit. I suppose that what Marie helped me to do was to integrate my sexuality into my chosen life as a nun.

It is clear from the accounts of all the nuns with whom I spoke that being celibate is a part of religious women's sexuality, and that sexual feeling is entwined into their celibate practice.

It is clear from Sister Angela's account that the difference between sexual intimacy and sexual celibacy is less a matter of genital contact than that matter of *focus*. Sister Hana Zarinah, whose controversial definition I quoted earlier ('Celibacy begins in the mind . . . I neither possess nor feel possessed'), pointed to freedom and autonomy as the basis of celibacy. Emotional or emotional and physical involvement can lead to possession, thence to lack of freedom. One woman clarified this further by suggesting that to be celibate you needed to be 'psychically free'.

Sister Angela bore this out when she said that she and the younger nun Marie 'began to focus on each other. That was the worst (although at the time it seemed the best); that focus on each other.' Later in her story, Sister Angela said that during the sexually intimate times with Marie she felt 'possessed'. Sexual possession it seems cannot be a part of the life of a celibate (religious) woman.

It is passion without possession which is sought through celibacy.

From *Women, Celibacy and Passion*, published by André Deutsch.

# NADEZHDA MANDELSTAM
## *Last Letter*

Nadezhda Mandelstam met her husband, the poet Osip Mandelstam, in May 1919. In May 1938 she watched as Stalin's
secret police took him away in a truck, never to be seen
again.

This letter was never read by the person it is addressed to. It is
written on two sheets of very poor paper. Millions of women
wrote such letters – to their husbands, sons, brothers, fathers,
or simply to sweethearts. But next to none of them have been
preserved. If such things ever survived here, it could only be
owing to chance, or a miracle. My letter still exists by chance.
I wrote it in October 1938, and in January I learned that M.
was dead. It was thrown into a trunk with other papers and
lay there for nearly thirty years. I came across it the last time I
went through all my papers, gladdened by every scrap of
something that had survived, and lamenting all the huge,
irreparable losses. I read it not at once, but only several years
later. When I did, I thought of all the other women who
shared my fate.

22/10(38)

Osia, my beloved, faraway sweetheart!

I have no words, my darling, to write this letter that you
may never read, perhaps. I am writing it into empty space.
Perhaps you will come back and not find me here. Then
this will be all you have left to remember me by.

Osia, what a joy it was living together like children – all
our squabbles and arguments, the games we played, and our
love. Now I do not even look at the sky. If I see a cloud,
who can I show it to?

Remember the way we brought back provisions to make

our poor feasts in all the places where we pitched out tent
like nomads? Remember the good taste of bread when we
got it by a miracle and ate it together? And our last winter
in Voronezh. Our happy poverty, and the poetry you
wrote. I remember the time we were coming back once
from the baths, when we bought some eggs or sausage, and
a cart went by loaded with hay. It was still cold and I was
freezing in my short jacket (but nothing like what we must
suffer now: I know how cold you are). That day comes
back to me now. I understand so clearly, and ache from the
pain of it, that those winter days with all their troubles
were the greatest and last happiness to be granted us in life.

My every thought is about you. My every tear and every
smile is for you. I bless every day and every hour of our
bitter life together, my sweetheart, my companion, my
blind guide in life.

Like two blind puppies, we were, nuzzling each other
and feeling so good together. And how fevered your poor
head was, and how madly we frittered away the days of our
life. What joy it was, and how we always knew what joy it
was.

Life can last so long. How hard and long for each of us
to die alone. Can this fate be for us who are inseparable?
Puppies and children, did we deserve this? Did you deserve
this, my angel? Everything goes on as before. I know
nothing. Yet I know everything — each day and hour of
your life are plain and clear to me as in a delirium.

You came to me every night in my sleep, and I kept
asking what had happened, but you did not reply.

In my last dream I was buying food for you in a filthy
hotel restaurant. The people with me were total strangers.
When I had bought it, I realised I did not know where to
take it, because I do not know where you are.

When I woke up, I said to Shura: 'Osia is dead.' I do not
know whether you are still alive, but from the time of that
dream, I have lost track of you. I do not know where you
are. Will you hear me? Do you know how much I love
you? I could never tell you how much I love you. I cannot

tell you even now. I speak only to you, only to you. You are with me always, and I who was such a wild and angry one and never learned to weep simple tears — now I weep and weep and weep.

It's me: Nadia. Where are you?

Farewell.

Nadia.

From *Hope Abandoned*, published by Collins Harvill.

# SHEILA JEFFREYS

## From *The Lesbian Heresy: A Feminist Perspective on the Lesbian Sexual Revolution*

This paper was written in 1984, when lesbian sadomasochism first became a concern in the British radical lesbian feminist community. Sheila Jeffreys is a radical feminist who has been at the forefront of lesbian feminist objections to sadomasochism, and the article from which these extracts have been taken has become a landmark text.

### SADOMASOCHISM: THE EROTIC CULT OF FASCISM

I became aware of the links between sadomasochism and fascism in 1981 when I visited Amsterdam from my home in London to attend the women's festival. An important, if not the main, theme of the festival was sadomasochism. Women at the Amsterdam festival demonstrated S/M scenarios, eg a male-to-constructed female transsexual whipping a woman, both dressed in fetishistic 'feminine' clothing and black leather. Quite a number of women at the festival were dressed in black leather and some were on collars and leads being led around by other women. The promotional workshops for S/M argued from the basis of personal freedom for sexual minorities. The promoters argued that S/M was basically a private affair, though S/M practitioners had to 'come out' because they were oppressed by prejudice and discrimination against their preferred sexual practice.

In the same week as the festival took place the first fascist member of parliament was elected in Amsterdam since the war. There were street fights that weekend in which fascists celebrated by beating up members of Amsterdam's immigrant population, and a telephone tree had to be operated to get anti-fascists to different parts of the town to resist the racist violence. The Amsterdam feminists who told me of the violence and the election triumph did not see any connection between the increase in fascism and the promotion of S/M as a sexual practice. They accepted that S/M was simply a personal matter. I was not convinced. A main Amsterdam police station was in the same street as the building, the Melkweg, in which the festival took place. Outside the festival building there was a massive wall poster of a full-length naked woman with her hands tied behind her. The slave woman appeared opposite the police station. She did not to me represent a symbol of defiance. It seemed likely that S/M, the police, a burgeoning fascist threat, the teenage boys who threw stones at myself and my lover for holding hands a street away from the festival, had a great deal in common . . .

The erotic roots of fascism lie in the way in which sexuality under male supremacy is structured in individuals. Because western male supremacy encourages us to experience sexuality as an immensely powerful and nigh uncontrollable force, the erotic aspect of fascism has great significance. We do not learn to express ourselves sexually in a world of equal, loving relationships. Women and men are born into the heterosexual system of male dominance and female submission. This holds true whether or not we are able to escape sufficiently to love women. Childhood sexuality is constructed through interaction with aggressive boys pulling girls' knickers down and through sexual abuse and exploitation by adult men. The models we are offered of female sexuality are of passivity and submission. We are taught to respond sexually to aggressive male overtures. Many lesbians have difficulty learning the correct female response to submissive sexual docility to men, but never the less we do not easily emerge unscathed from the construction of female sexuality around sadomasochism. Where we live under oppression and where there is virtually no escape for us, at least until we reach an advanced age, toward egalitarian relationships in which we take sexual initiatives, we have little alternative but to take pleasure from our oppression. The most common response is to eroticise our powerlessness in masochism. For some women who see this as too 'effeminate' the role of humiliating women can be eroticised in sadism – the models for this in a woman-hating culture are everywhere.

Lesbians and gay men suffer particular pressures which can lead to the possession of a sexuality constructed around sado-masochism. As a result of heterosexism and anti-lesbianism, we have often grown up hating ourselves and particularly our sexuality. It is hard for us to build for ourselves a sexuality that is positive, egalitarian and free from S/M overtones. Some lesbians and gay men know no other sexuality than that of sadomasochistic fantasies which influence their practice, though they may studiously avoid acting out S/M ritual. Any challenge to sadomasochism is felt by some lesbians and gay men as a serious threat. They see themselves as having no sexual practice at all if they have to abandon that which is based on eroticising oppression. But there lies, in our very understanding that sexuality is something constructed and not given, a message of hope. We can reconstruct. There is every ground for optimism. Some lesbians and gay men are very little affected by S/M, and are able to practise a different kind of sexuality. Even those of us who do know the extent of S/M influence in our lives usually have experienced moments of unusual sexual intensity and pleasure which have not involved fantasised dominance and submission to any degree. In all of us are the seeds of change. We can seek to maximise positive sexuality instead of maximising the negative sexuality of S/M.

The triggers to a sexual response built around masochism are the symbols of power and authority. Particularly powerful symbols are those which represent abusive, cruel and arbitrary power and authority, the whip is a more powerful symbol than the prefect's badge. The trappings and rituals of fascism are perfect symbols for the purpose. Uniforms, marches, swastikas, portraits of Hitler, authoritarian speechmaking are erotic triggers. The sadists in the National Front are stimu-lated by repeated viewing of videos of German nazi marches and parades. All the paraphernalia of fascism is calculated to draw a powerful erotic response from those whose sexuality has been formed under male supremacy and modelled on sadomasochism. That is most of us.

It is the capacity to be attracted to nazism that numbs the response of outrage that many people might otherwise feel toward it. The construction of S/M sexuality is a mighty clever ploy for the oppressor. Our resistance is undermined in our very guts if our response to the torture of others or to the trappings of militarism is erotic rather than politically indignant. It is very hard to fight what turns you on. This is a problem which feminists fighting porn have already recognised and understood. It feels humiliating and paralysing to be turned on by the very degradation of women that you wish to challenge. The only way to fight is to turn that pain into anger. We are not to blame for the way our sexuality is constructed, though we have total responsibility for how we choose to act on it. We have the right to be furious and to direct our pain into attacking the porn merchants, the porn apologists (and they include, unfortunately, S/M dykes), the porn buyers and consumers. It's hard but we have to understand that the images and messages – of women being objects, tortured, used and abused – that influence our own sexual response are meant to paralyse us. We cannot afford to be weakened by these images but must share our feelings and build our rage.

As with sexism, the trappings of fascism and even its practice can be turn-ons not just for the oppressor but for his victims. Edmund White, US gay novelist, interviewed a couple of gay men who were into wearing police uniforms in his book *States of Desire: Travels in Gay America*. He explained that there was a bar staffed with gay men in police uniforms in which the customers included gay men dressed as cops and real life policemen. This tragic and degrading flirtation with oppression had alarming implications. One cop lookalike, when arrested later outside the bar, spent his time entranced by the policeman's boots. Another who was arrested and beaten up could speak of nothing but his infatuation for his tormentor.[1]

S/M promoters constantly stress that S/M is 'only fantasy' and bears no relation to reality. This is a comforting illusion. What is ritual today can be reality tomorrow. The promotion of S/M and its imagery will ensure that it will be more and more difficult in the future for some lesbians and gay men, perhaps for all those who use the gay social scene, which is flooded with S/M imagery, to be purely angry and in no sense erotically aroused by the imagery of real life, practising fascists, policemen, and thugs. I think it is important that we are able to distinguish fascist threats accurately and fight them clearly. I do not want to think that, when tanks and marching boots and swastikas pass by in a real fascist coup, the gay population will be experiencing a thud of erotic desire which immobilises us.

From *The Lesbian Heresy: A Feminist Perspective on the Lesbian Sexual Revolution* by Sheila Jeffreys, published by The Women's Press.

# SAL AND ANNE
*Stepping Out*

## SAL'S STORY

The year I turned seven my world changed. I left home to go to a special school and discovered I was a person with a disability and a new vocabulary to describe myself.

I was born partially sighted due to a hereditary condition known as ocular albinoism, made worse by the fact that my retinas were burnt when I was given pure oxygen a few hours after birth. My uncle made the discovery by passing a lighted match in front of my eyes; there wasn't a flicker. There followed years of visits to specialists, something I stopped at eighteen. No more bloody professionals.

Until I was seven I had just felt different. I was the kid who had hair as white as ice-cream, the kid you gave specific directions to – 'I'm in the kitchen by the fridge' – the kid who hard large black letters on her lunch box. I had the easiest seat to find in my classroom, my clothes-peg was at the end of the row, no one would remove furniture or leave things lying around without telling me, and no one would respond to me by nodding their heads. I was the kid who always had the most bruises.

At seven, however, I became a problem because I wasn't learning like the rest of my class. So the professionals stepped in, and in April 1969 I began a new life at the National Institute for the Blind and the Partially Sighted unit at Thomas Street Primary School in Perth, Western Australia, 130 miles from my parents' farm. After Thomas Street I moved on to Sutherland Street. I learned braille and in my last year, aged thirteen, discovered a magnifying glass, something which was not encouraged. Over the next six years I made up for never having been able to read a printed book by cramming in the whole range, from baby books, through children's books and teenage books to adult reading.

At fourteen I moved back home. I was two years behind in school and behaviour, but my body was well into puberty. I had little sexual awareness as far as fantasies or feelings went, but I did know about sex or at least about how babies were conceived, though I didn't quite believe that anybody would be willing to do it. Being at home full-time meant I lost the privileges that went with coming home only occasionally. Things didn't go my way so easily and my parents and I began to experience the trauma of adolescence. My former classmates were now two years above me, but I had kept in touch with some of them and basically knew my way around. I was able to hold my own in class and over time was accepted.

The year I turned sixteen I fell in love with Jane, though at the time I could never have used those words to describe my feelings. We were in the same year and spent time together during breaks, after school and at weekends. We frequently stayed at each other's houses and would always sleep in the same bed, though we made the pretence of having slept apart as we knew for some reason we shouldn't. Nothing sexual happened between us.

Meanwhile, I began to put my energies into pretending that Clay was the person of the moment, while Jane really did fall in love – with James, a teacher. I spent this time being awfully cross and not quite knowing why, a situation I resolved in part by deciding to go away to school to do my A level equivalents at the Methodist Ladies College in Perth. After the relative familiarity of a school and classmates I had known since early childhood, the stress of being 'different' began to build up again. I had one good friend at that time – also someone who didn't quite fit because she was Asian. I felt glad no longer to be at a co-ed school and to be away from home but didn't think things through much further. It was a pattern of burying my feelings that continued as I grew older.

In 1982 I started a psychology degree. What became

important at this time was personal growth and establishing myself as an independent person. Against the pleas of my mother and sisters, my father agreed to lend me the money to buy a bicycle, which enabled me to go further than college for support. At the same time I began to see myself as having a disability and to question society's part in that. And I started to become aware of myself as a sexual being. Someone had begun to talk about lesbianism, which fitted a vague idea I had about myself but wasn't ready to confront: until now I had pretty much ignored what sexual feelings I'd had.

In May 1983, after having been ill for a couple of months and losing an extraordinary amount of weight, my world fell apart. I felt physically weak and emotionally unable to deal with all the puzzles my mind was coming up with. So I ran. I took six months off, travelling around Australia and thinking as little as possible, ignoring my mind screaming for answers.

The following year I was offered a place on the speech and hearing pathology course I had originally applied for, and felt obliged to accept. Later in the same year I had a bicycle accident, which acted like a catalyst in forcing me to think. For the first time, I thought about who I was and who I wanted to be. I rejected the image forced on me by my parents of a good girl who was going to get a good job. I also decided that at twenty-two it was about time I got rid of my virginity and began to find out about sex by discussing it with anyone who would listen, and by reading. A couple of years previously, I had found myself intensely attracted to a bloke called Chris, but unfortunately I had been unable to separate my sexual feelings from an idealised notion of romantic love and he got scared: neither of us was ready to say *it's only lust, so let's get down to it*. This time I wasn't going to make the same mistake, so I found a nice bloke, decided he was *it*, and made sure I stated clearly what I wanted. It was okay, safe, fun, and lasted for three weeks. It gave me yet more confidence: I rejected the idea that being fat was bad and that having a disability was my problem.

On 30 November 1984 I walked into a travel agency and bought a ticket to England. I arrived on 15 January 1985; it was snowing and I knew no one. That year I got my first real job, working for the Youth Hostels Association, and had my first 'real' relationship, which grew out of a good working relationship, a shared history in Australia, and a need in David to rescue someone. It lasted on and off for seven months. That same year I also came out as a lesbian. I was working on the Isle of Wight as an assistant warden and my decision was sparked off by two women who turned up at the hostel one weekend. Something inside me went *wow*, and that was it: I was out and so was David. Being so far away from my family, it was possible not to feel guilty. It also helped that my boss was gay and he gave me a lot of support.

In 1986 I came back to London to work for Feminist Audio Books, a tape library of feminist and lesbian material for blind and partially sighted women. My crude understanding of disability politics became polished and I began a series of jobs in equal opportunities. I had different lovers, lived in different places and learnt to live with my thoughts. I remember admitting to myself and to a close friend that I would probably only have a relationship with a disabled woman if she was partially sighted – a hard one to come to terms with, as I saw myself as pretty right on. Later that year I went to a benefit and was bowled over by a woman. It was lust at first sight and out flew my vow of a period of celibacy. She happened to be a wheelchair user.

As soon as I saw Anne I started to ask friends who she was. Finally someone introduced me. I was in lust, and what registered more than the fact that this woman was sitting in a wheelchair was that she looked young. My resolve of celibacy was ebbing away as I set out to make an impression.

I left the benefit with a kiss and her phone number and it took me two days to pluck up courage to phone her. My reluctance had very little to do with her being a wheelchair user and all to do with my fear of being rejected. We had a brief conversation and agreed to meet the following Saturday, and here we are, two and a bit years later.

I can remember thinking about what we would be up

against if we got into a relationship. My thoughts had little to do with how we would make love and a lot to do with where we would go out. Anne couldn't come to my house and what would we do if we were invited to a party and it was inaccessible? I blocked out a lot of my thoughts, and was outraged with friends who voiced the same anxieties.

The beginning was fun. We spent most of our time in bed and friends, family, home and work were neglected. Slowly a pattern began to form in which I was spending most of my time with Anne at her place, very little at home and just enough at work to get paid. What was going on? Why weren't we going anywhere? We spent a lot of time reassuring each other that staying home was okay. It gave us time to talk and we found out that we shared a lot of common experiences about growing up as disabled people. We also spent a lot of time avoiding issues that were beginning to raise their ugly heads. We skirted around my growing anger about never being at home and Anne never being able to come home with me. We avoided discussions about not going out and about being invited to parties that were inaccessible.

One of the things that I have discovered through being with Anne is the importance of being able to go out to the theatre, cinema, exhibitions, together. For me it's about sharing and finding common ground. As our relationship progressed I began to suggest more and more things, but however varied my ideas were they met with little enthusiasm.

I have been given the answers to Anne's reluctance mostly through the experience of going out itself. For example, earlier this year we decided to go to see a film at the Barbican. I rang and got a yes to all my questions about access. The cab we'd booked (which turned up late, so we missed the six o'clock screening we'd planned for and were left with the problem of having to rearrange our return journey) dropped us at the front entrance, where we were faced with a glorious view of the complex from the top of several flights of stairs. How to get down was solved by a man who came up to see what we wanted and then disappeared to get the key to the stair lift. He explained that to get to the cinema we should use the staff lift to level five and then go outside to another lift which would take us to level nine. He added that there were no facilities up there, so if we wanted coffee or a drink we should do that first.

After coffee on level five, a drink on level six and the toilet on level one it was back to level five, only to find that the concourse area had been locked and our way blocked. The response to our question about how to get to level nine was 'take the lift to level eight and walk' – you could have given the man a medal for not noticing that Anne was a wheelchair user. We finally found ourselves following a top security man, who led us up lifts and down corridors, assuring us all the time that the access was fine.

Once on the right level, I left Anne sitting by the door and went to buy tickets. Now it was the usherette's turn to get into a tizz: Anne became invisible and I was told to push her in last; I could sit at the back. Secure in the knowledge that we were going to be able to get into the film, we decided to use the remaining spare time to try to arrange a cab home, which meant back to level three. When I asked the usherette to explain to Anne how to get there as giving me visual directions is useless, she said she would write it down. At this point we began to wonder if we shouldn't just give up and go home.

We stayed. Anne sat in her wheelchair at the back and I was told to sit behind her, to the right. This was no good because I need to be able to ask questions as I find it difficult to recognize faces, which means by the time I've sorted out who's who the film is over. I asked for a chair so I could sit beside her and was refused because of fire regulations, so I got our coats and sat on the floor.

It's not an unusual experience whenever we go anywhere new for me to have a queasy feeling in my stomach about whether the place will really be accessible. If it is, the relief is tremendous. Often I am put into a position in which my disability is forgotten: I am treated as Anne's carer, the one with all my faculties, while Anne is ignored.

113

Anne and I now live together and experience the same problems as other people who live together. We are managing to do a lot more and Anne, to her credit, allows herself to be hauled up and down flights of steps by me. We have recently succeeded in having a holiday in Hong Kong and the Philippines, and despite the usual hassles (a hotel that had steps up to the entrance and no way of getting to the bathroom) we coped and had a good time. We have learnt that each of us experiences indignity and hurt from such situations but the important thing is not to give up, not to take it out on each other, and to keep trying to live life the way we want to.

## ANNE'S STORY

I was fifteen months old when arthritis came into my life. My left knee and the little finger of my right hand were the first joints affected. By 1969, when I was two, my left leg had a splint that was removed only when I had a bath, or to exercise. My earliest memories include realising I had a bad leg and being told I was 'special' because of it. I stopped wearing that splint full time when I was three or four.

On the one hand my family encouraged me to be a 'normal' kid, even down to the beatings I would get if I was naughty; on the other they were overprotective. My mother wouldn't allow me to cross the road on my own until I was fifteen or sixteen, while my brothers, especially the younger one, acted like minders. But my father and I always got on very well. He never hid the fact that I was his favourite, and I never hid the fact that I milked it.

Sex and sexuality weren't serious questions until, at the age of eleven, I was sent to boarding school. The school was for kids with physical disabilities: you know, one of those 'special schools'. The year I started, some of the brighter members of the Board decided it should become a co-ed set up. It was obvious that nobody expected disabled kids to get up to anything of a sexual nature, but they couldn't have been more wrong. They had manufactured a promiscuous society. Within a short space of time I had my first boyfriend.

I was very curious about sex with boys and forgot the sexual fantasies I'd had about women. A vivid memory from my childhood is finding a pile of porn mags in my brother's bedroom when I was about eight. I would go and look at them whenever I could: it was a strange experience because although I was totally enthralled by the pictures, I can remember thinking that women's genitals were ugly, and I was sure I didn't want to grow up looking like that. In retrospect, I recognise I felt sexual, though I didn't understand that at the time and hadn't yet discovered masturbation. I wanted to be a boy and grow up to be a man.

But that all went by the wayside in my first year at school. I had a number of boyfriends and soon began to have sex. I hadn't started my periods so pregnancy was not a problem, which is just as well, because as a Catholic the rhythm method was the only form of contraception I knew. During my first sexual experiences my biggest worry was guilt. I didn't want my mother to find out; I was sure the shock would be too much for her. I was convinced I was in love with everyone I went out with, but I think now that this was an excuse to make it all seem okay.

At the end of my first year I had to go into the hospital I had been attending since I was eight for an assessment. When I went into that hospital I was twelve and walking; when I came out: I was thirteen and in a wheelchair. I had been able to walk, run and even ride a bike, but because my posture wasn't good it was decided to operate on my hips. The right hip was done first and it passed without too many problems.

After a boring and painful three months in bed I was given the choice of having my left hip done or starting to walk on my right leg. I chose to start walking, but my physiotherapist encouraged me to change my mind and so I had my left hip done. Even though all the relevant tests were carried out and the doctors knew I had a urine infection, they performed the operation, without antibiotics. Shortly afterwards I started to become very ill, so ill I wished I was dead. I became totally dehydrated and my body was full of poison because my kidneys had failed. Eventually, when I was very nearly dead, it was decided that a drip should be put in my arm and antibiotics given intravenously. I recovered quite quickly, though the delay in starting physiotherapy for my hip meant that it never became strong or mobile enough again. The experience left me with a lot to think about.

As time went on and I was still in hospital I went into a deep depression. I was on a ward for teenage girls and women with arthritis and my only good memories of that time are of the other patients. When I left it was with a feeling that I had discovered true friendship.

I had a week at home and then it was back to school. I fell back into the old routine and started going out with boys again, only this time I didn't waste any emotion, I just got what I wanted out of it. In any relationship the biggest discussion would be where we would go to 'have a bit' – in fact, this was usually the *only* thing we talked about. More often than not we managed – for example, with one particular boy I would go over to the building site that later became the sixth form hostel. The relationships were all heterosexual and I heard of only two cases in which a boy (never any girls) tried it on with another boy.

Of the relationships I had at school, all but one was physical. That one relationship lasted for a year and in the whole time he only gave me two pecks on the cheek. Yet because I was emotionally involved, it was the most important of all. We talked to each other, went for walks, had fun and generally acted like a couple. I was aware that something was missing from my other relationships, but I put it down to the fact that my emotions were all spent, and that I wasn't a very emotional person anyway. In retrospect, I think this was all a big excuse to get away from the fact that it was difficult for me to relate emotionally to the opposite sex.

When we were about fifteen all the haemophiliac boys at the school, of which there was a high percentage, started to use condoms whenever they had sex. I thought how responsible they were being and admired them. It wasn't until I left that I discovered that they had all contracted HIV from the factorate they had to use when they had bleeds. No one else at the school was told; instead, a ban was slapped on sex. Of course it didn't stop us at all, in fact it only encouraged us further. Since leaving school I've heard a lot of these boys have developed Aids and died.

At around this time I decided not to have any more boy-friends because I realised I needed to think and wanted to spend more time on my own. Sexuality was something I had to think about seriously. I was becoming more and more aware of my sexual preference for women and it scared the shit out of me. I had sexual dreams about women that I would try to push out of my mind when I woke up. I was also finding it more and more difficult to control my sexual fantasies about women — something I had had from the age of ten or eleven and had tried to stop. In my last year at school my hatred of 'queers' and 'poofs' took up a lot of my emotional and mental energy, though I now know that all it did was to confirm to people who knew me that I was a lesbian. I kept telling myself that as long as I still fancied boys it must be all right.

I also thought a lot about why we were all at it like rabbits — not just sex but smoking and other things besides. It came to me that I did these things because it was 'normal', that it felt important to keep up with other kids who didn't have disabilities. I became aware of oppression and how the school staff tried to suppress our sexuality. I remembered a time in the hospital when I was told by the sister to stop seeing a boy from the teenage boys' ward. The relationship hadn't been much more than a friendship, but I realise that I had been told to stop because I had a disability.

I began to hate the school even more once I realised what it stood for. There we were, disabled kids in a convenient corner in the middle of nowhere. Why weren't we at home? Our parents had been convinced it was the best place for us. Why? I was too young and inexperienced to work it out, but I knew I was mightily pissed off. I became a very angry and bitter young person. It wasn't until some years later that I realised this was the beginning of my political awakening. I wish I could have used it then in the way I can use it now.

Hospital and school had institutionalised me; at home I felt lonely and alienated, confused and terribly insecure. I decided I was going to need privacy and plenty of time on my own, so at seventeen, before I left school, I put myself on a council housing waiting list. I knew that I needed to establish a base for myself, somewhere where I could have the privacy I craved to discover my identity. I left school when I was nearly eighteen and was able to move into my own place two years later. The freedom and privacy overwhelmed me at first, but it did ultimately have a calming effect; and I became less highly strung than I had been in my teenage years.

Shortly after moving I started coming out to friends as bisexual, which seemed easier than admitting to being a lesbian. I decided I wouldn't just come out, but that I would sound people out first. I was pleased with the general response, which tended to be 'so what?' In fact, despite my attempts to hide it, most people had sussed it already. I was confused because I still felt physically attracted to men. But the point I had been missing was what whereas with men it was physical but not emotional, with women it was both. By twenty-one I was no longer confused. I knew that to be lesbian was natural to me, and was okay.

When I had just turned twenty-two I met, through some work I was doing, an 'out' lesbian. She asked me directly if I was a dyke. I responded by saying I was a bit of both. She was a professional counsellor and I decided to have some counselling sessions. At the time I was still having sex with men but I desperately wanted to come out as a lesbian and knew I couldn't on my own. Through the counselling sessions we became friends and she encouraged me to go out. I had known about pubs and clubs for some time but I hadn't gone to any because I had no one to go with. Having a disability made me self-conscious, and I so desperately wanted to fit in. After all, I had waited so long. The first women-only event I went out to was a benefit for disabled women. I knew it would be accessible and I had the support of friends. It was here I met Sal, my girlfriend. Before I met her I had never had sex with another woman. I had had an emotional but not a physical involvement with someone, but I was nineteen and couldn't handle it, so I just let it fall through. About a year later I had what I can only call 'a bit' with another young woman. It was experimental on both our parts and basically we just kissed and touched each other from the waist up. Sal is still the only woman I've had sex with. We're still together.

My account of our first meeting isn't as romantic as Sal's. I hadn't been 'out' for long and as it was the first time I'd been to a women–only event I was in a state of awe at the number of dykes around me. One thing for sure was that I was a single dyke, and that I was convinced I would stay that way for a long time. After all, no one meets a partner the first time they go to a women–only event, and, of course, I was a wheelchair user and past experience had taught me that disabled people aren't considered to have any form of sexuality. It wasn't until the end of the evening, when Sal asked for my phone number, that I realised she was interested. A couple of days later she contacted me and we arranged to meet the following weekend. Obviously we had to meet somewhere that was accessible and so straight away the pattern of the relationship was set.

Like most new relationships there followed a honeymoon period where physically we learned so much about each other. During this time we had many intimate conversations about each other's childhood and past experiences. It soon became clear that we had a lot in common. I still felt curious about whether, in the beginning, Sal had wondered how, or even if, I could have sex. A little while into the relationship I asked her about this. She answered by saying it had never been an issue for her; in fact the opposite was true, and she couldn't wait to get into bed with me. Needless to say I was pleased by her answer.

The honeymoon started coming to an end two to three months after we met. The major part of that time had been spent in bed. For me it had been great, and relaxing. The strain for Sal, however, had started to show. She was not only physically tired, but mentally and emotionally too. Her work was suffering because she wasn't getting enough sleep. Also, her friends seemed to be getting upset because of the amount of time she spent at my place. I can remember thinking how unfair they were being – wasn't it obvious that she had to come to my place because I couldn't get into hers? It seemed to take a long time for some of Sal's friends to realise why she had to come to my place and not vice versa. These things became issues between us.

We agreed to sit down and discuss how we were going to handle the situation. Sal needed more sleep, which meant less sex. We had a number of arguments over it and grudgingly I agreed that she needed more rest than she had been getting. Once the novelty of the relationship had worn off, I felt embarrassed about my behaviour at that time.

The other issue was the attitude of her friends, some of whom had what I perceived as a stubborn lack of understanding. I was angry and was convinced they resented and disliked me; they made clear the fact that my disability was a problem for them. One of the biggest decisions we made was that if we were invited to a party it had to be accessible, otherwise neither of us would go. I realised then how committed Sal was to our relationship.

We'd been seeing each other for seven months when we decided to live together. Up to that point whenever Sal came round we would stay in. It wasn't that I was content to do so; it was just easier. Not surprisingly Sal started to get restless with this arrangement. Why didn't we go anywhere or do anything? It was my turn to feel pressured. I tried to explain the difficulties I'd had as a wheelchair user whenever I'd gone out in the past. All my experiences had made me apathetic. Also, as a wheelchair user the choice of places to go (especially in the lesbian and gay sector) is minimal. Finding an accessible venue or pub or club is difficult enough, but the problems don't stop there. One of the worst things is toilets. I've lost count of the number of times I've contacted somewhere to find out the access details, been reassured that there is full access, and then found I couldn't use the toilet. It means either I don't drink anything, or (if I happen to be with someone) I sneak outside to the nearest alley or dark corner. It usually ends with a shorter than expected time out and a desperate journey home. And then there's transport. It does tend to spoil a night out when at one in the morning you find yourself waiting for a mini-cab to turn up, knowing that it could be another hour before it does so.

For a long time I was adamant that going out was too much trouble for me but that if it was important to Sal she should go with friends or on her own. Finally she persuaded me. It wasn't an easy or spontaneous process: we always had to plan where we went some time in advance and if things went wrong, always through no fault of our own, we would argue. I felt as if she blamed me because without me she wouldn't have had the problems; I blamed her for making me go out in the first place. It hasn't been like that every time, in fact the bad experiences don't outnumber the good and exciting ones. We have Sal's persistence and optimism to thank for that, and I have to admit that I am more often than not grateful for it. We have reached a stage now where we don't blame each other if a venue is not accessible. It has also made a huge difference that I passed my driving test earlier in the year and now that we've got a car it's our decision when we go out and when we come home. There are times now when it's me who has to badger Sal out of the door.

Sal and I have had many personal problems in our relation-ship – who doesn't? But what of all the other problems we've had to deal with as well? I mean the problems this society has caused us – the physical barriers of inaccessibility, the patronising and often hostile attitude of some non-disabled people. All this has made it harder for us. We are disabled people having a relationship in a non-disabled world.

It's tough for us but we're strong stuff, we've made it work and we're still making it work. We know that each other and our relationship are worth fighting for.

---

From *Women Talk Sex*, edited by Pearlie McNeill, Bea Freeman and Jenny Newman, published by Scarlet Press.

# ROBERTA MORRIS

## *A Feminist Ovary Goes Its Own Way*
### (for Dr Fay Weisberg and Dr Caroline Bennett)

Our sexuality is our way of being in the world. I go on tour to convince women that our bodies are friendly, that we don't exist as the counterpart of male intellectual and spiritual purity. Female sexuality exists apart from men's fears and temptations. This is the lecture I deliver, the poems and stories I write: Celebrate; dance. I celebrate myself. I dance. I paint this happy face on female sexuality and then my ovary erupts, dumping half my blood into my abdomen, and I feel a little silly.

With many female diseases there is an identifiable enemy. Poor nutrition. Dangerous birth-control devices. Since cervical and breast tissue absorb nasty chemicals, pollution is probably the villain in the rise of female cancers. Genetically programmed female tissue plays housewife, sweeping up nuclear dust. But this doesn't explain why my happy little ovary, from whence came Andrea and Nathaniel, turns mean.

The doctor, like a good mother separating two quarrelling children, does not lay blame but plucks up my ovary and sends me to my room. My ovary remains in OR.

Now where did they put it? I imagine the obstetrical ward's OR garbage, a deconstructed image of the female reproductive system that is featured on the ward walls. A Cubist sculptor with a taste for the baroque might do it justice, a mound of uteruses, ovaries, placenta, pieces of human reproduction piled high.

An amputee continues to feel the missing limb as a ghost appendage, just as I imagine my ovary whistles at me from atop the garbage heap, 'Hey cutie, but didn't we have a grand time?'

---

From *Eating Apples: Knowing Women's Lives*, edited by Caterina Edwards and Kay Stewart, published by NeWest Press

# ZORA NEALE HURSTON
## *Formulae of Hoodoo Doctors*

### TO MAKE PEOPLE LOVE YOU

Take nine lumps of starch, nine of sugar, nine teaspoons of steel dust. Wet it all with Jockey Club cologne. Take nine pieces of ribbon, blue, red or yellow. Take a dessertspoonful and put it on a piece of ribbon and tie it in a bag. As each fold is gathered together call his name. As you wrap it with yellow thread call his name till you finish. Make nine bags and place them under a rug, behind an armoire, under a step or over a door. They will love you and give you everything they can get. Distance makes no difference. Your mind is talking to his mind and nothing beats that.

### TO BREAK UP A LOVE AFFAIR

Take nine needles, break each needle in three pieces. Write each person's name three times on paper. Write one name backwards and one forwards and lay the broken needles on the paper. Take five black candles, four red and three green.

Tie a string across the door from it, suspend a large candle upside down. It will hang low on the door; burn one each day for one hour. If you burn your first in the daytime, keep on in the day; if at night, continue at night. A tin plate with paper and needles in it must be placed to catch wax in.

When the ninth day is finished, go out into the street and get some white or black dog dung. A dog only drops his dung in the street when he is running and barking, and whoever you curse will run and bark likewise. Put it in a bag with the paper and carry it to running water, and one of the parties will leave town.

---

From *Mules and Men*, published by HarperCollins.

# Notes

From *Women Like Us* by Marie, pages 40–43.

1. *Sappho* magazine was formed after the collapse of *Arena 3* in 1971. Women continued to meet in the Museum Tavern, Museum St, London and in 1972 the first copy of the lesbian feminist magazine, *Sappho*, appeared. Unlike *Arena 3* it was produced by a collective who then went on to organise discos and meetings. The magazine folded in December 1981 and the discos finished in 1982.

2. Older Lesbian Network, c/o Wesley House, 4 Wild Court, London WC2B 5AU.

*Really Being in Love Means Wanting to Live in a Different World* by Lucy Goodison, pages 59–81.

1. The leaflet, headed 'Everything tends to reduce lovers to objects', is marked BIB 2, bubble CPP – bm.

2. This lack of discussion of the subject is pointed out by Daphne Davis, 'Falling in Love again', *Red Rag, A Magazine of Women's Liberation*, No. 13, p. 12. Elizabeth Wilson also notes with regret the way that socialism and feminism have neglected romance in 'Fruits of Passion', *City Limits*, No. 74, March 1983.

3. This point is expressed more fully by Davis, *op. cit.*, pp. 12, 13.

4. From Alison Buckley 'For Tasha', in *Art and Feminism*, Laurieston Hall, 1977.

5. Rosie Boycott, 'Falling in love again', *Honey*, IPC Magazines, 1982. The article is a detailed personal account of the start of an intense love affair.

6. Marge Piercy, *Small Changes*, Fawcett Publications, Greenwich, Conn. 1974, p. 193.

7. *ibid.*, pp. 194, 195.

8. *Ink in Love: Exploding the Romantic Myth*, Ink, No. 29, 21 February 1972, p. 12.

9. This is one of a number of personal accounts by women which for reasons of privacy I am leaving anonymous. I am indebted to a number of other women who have discussed their experiences with me, have read this piece and expressed encouragement and valuable disagreements, as well as giving helpful contributions and suggestions

about changes. In particular I would like to thank Sue Cartledge, Inga Czudnochowski, Marie Maguire, Jo Ryan and Stef Pixner.

10. Again, this point is made by Davis, *op. cit.*, p. 13.

11. Buckley, *op. cit.*

12. Piercy, *op. cit.*, p. 195.

13. Erica Jong, *How to Save Your Own Life*, Panther Books, London, 1977, pp. 203, 204, 207, 208.

14. See note 9, above.

15. Piercy, *op. cit.*, p. 197.

16. Piercy, 'Burying blues for Janis', in Lucille Iverson and Kathryn Ruby (eds), *We Become New: Poems by Contemporary American Women*, Bantam Books, 1975, pp. 4–5.

17. *ibid.*

18. Slim, 'If I loved me half as much as I love you', in *Country Women*, issue 24, pp. 18–20.

19. Jong, *op. cit.*, p. 207.

20. *Ink in Love, op. cit.*, p. 8.

21. Frederick S. Perls, *Gestalt Therapy Verbatim*, Bantam Books, London, 1971, p. 10.

22. This point is made in Ralph Metzner, *Maps of Consciousness*, Collier Macmillan, London, 1971, p. 152. Showing that projection is not unique to this century, Stendhal discusses the same process under the term 'crystallisation'. See Stendhal, *Love*, trans. by Gilbert and Suzanne Sale, Penguin, Harmondsworth, 1975.

23. See Liz Greene, *Relating: An Astrological Guide to Living with others on a small Planet*, Coventure, London, 1976, pp. 149–50.

24. Raymond Durgnat, *Eros in the Cinema*, Marion Boyars, 1966.

25. Perls, *op. cit.*, p. 40.

26. Metzner, *op. cit.*, p. 152.

27. Jane Roberts, *The Nature of Personal Reality: A Seth Book*, Prentice-Hall, New Jersey, 1974, p. 382.

28. See Roberto Assagioli, *Psychosynthesis*, Turnstone Books, 1975, pp. 25–6.

29. Melanie Klein, *Envy and Gratitude and Other Works 1946–63*, Hogarth Press, 1963, p. 100.

30. Jane Rule, 'Homophobia and romantic love', in *Outlander: Stories and Essays*, The Naiad Press, Florida, 1981, p. 184.

31. Piercy, *Small Changes*, p. 211.

32. Jenny James, *Room to Breathe*, Coventure, London, 1975, p. 151.

33. See, for example, Dion Fortune, *The Esoteric Philosophy of Love and Marriage*, The Aquarian Press, Wellingborough, 1974, pp. 60–62.

34. Davis in *Red Rag, op cit.*, p. 13, makes this point and suggests that we may imagine we are in love when all we are feeling are sexual desires or hunger pangs.

35. See note 9, above.

36. For a fuller account of this theory, see David V Tansley, *Radionics and the Subtle Anatomy of Man*, Health Science Press, Devon, 1972.

37. For a brief account of this method, see Brian and Marita Snellgrove, *The Unseen Self*, Kirlian Aura Diagnosis, Carshalton, Surrey, 1979.

38. Béla Grunberger, 'Narcissism in female sexuality', in Janine Chasseguet-Smirgel, (ed), *Female Sexuality: New Psychoanalytic Views*, Virago, London, 1981, p. 71.

39. Alexander Lowen, *Bioenergetics*, Coventure, London, 1976, p. 67.

40. This term comes from the books of Carlos Castaneda. See, for example, the incident where Castaneda 'sees' the 'lines', in *Journey to Ixtlan*, Penguin, Harmondsworth, 1974, p. 267.

41. This idea is suggested by the Arica spiritual teachings.

42. Perls, for example, distinguishes 'confluence' from real contact which consists of the appreciation of differences. See *Gestalt Therapy Verbatim*, pp. 271–2.

43. As Davis points out in *Red Rag, op. cit.*, p. 12.

44. For many of the ideas in this passage, and particularly here, I am indebted to the therapeutic work of Jenner Roth in her sexuality workshops and in her individual therapy practice in London.

45. See note 44.

46. See note 44.

47. Rule, *op. cit.*, p. 185.

48. Slim, *op. cit.*, p. 20.

49. Gestalt therapy offers some simple and useful techniques for owning fantasies and projections by role-playing. See Sheila Ernst and Lucy Goodison, *In Our Own Hands*, The Women's Press, London, 1981, chs. 3, 6.

50. *Ink in Love, op. cit.*, p. 9.

51. See note 9, above.

52. *Ink in Love, op. cit.*, p. 12.

*Convent Girls and Impossible Passions* by Sally Cline, pages 82–98.

1. Jackie Bennett and Rosemary Forgan (eds) *There's Something About a Convent Girl*, (Virago, London, 1991, p. 37.

2. Carole Angier, *Jean Rhys*, André Deutsch, London, 1990, p. 25.

3. Jackie Bennett and Rosemary Forgan, *op. cit.*, p. 90.

4. Carole Angier, *op. cit.*, p. 25.

5. Jackie Bennett and Rosemary Forgan, *op. cit.*, p. 27.

6. D M Feldman, *Birth Control in Jewish Law*, (New York University Press, New York, 1968), in *Sex: Facts, Frauds and Follies*, Thomas Szasz Basil Blackwell, Oxford, 1981, p. 104.

7. *ibid.*, p. 110.
8. Polly Blue, 'A Time to Refrain from Embracing', in Linda Hurcombe (ed), *Sex and God*, Routledge and Kegan Paul, New York, 1987, pp. 69–70.

## From *The Lesbian Heresy: A Feminist Perspective on the Lesbian Sexual Revolution* by Sheila Jeffreys, pages 102–106.

1. Edmund White, *States of Desire: Travels in Gay America*, Dutton, New York, 1983. If anything, the use of real-life torment as a sexual turn-on has increased since White's observations. Recently a staff person at the Glad Day bookstore in Boston told me that Daniel P Mannix's *History of Torture*, Dell, New York, 1983, is the store's best seller.

# Contributors' Notes

**Jane Blue** received an MA in Creative Writing from the University of California at Davis, where she studied with Karl Shapiro and Sandra M Gilbert. Her work has appeared in many literary magazines, including *Calyx, Carolina Quarterly, Ironwood, Visions International*, and *The Prose Poem*. For many years she taught a workshop in Wellspring Women's Center in Sacramento; recently, she has been employed at Folsom Prison, a maximum security men's prison.

**Margery Brews** was a woman who lived in fifteenth-century Norfolk.

**Sally Cline** is a writer, mother, feminist and academic, and was for many years Co-Course Organiser for Women's Studies at Cambridge University. Her short stories have been published in the UK and Canada and, in addition to *Women, Celibacy and Passion*, she is the author of *Just Desserts: Women and Food* and (with Dale Spender) *Reflecting Men at Twice their Natural Size*.

**Sidonie Gabrielle Colette** was born in Burgundy in 1873 and died in Paris in 1954.

She began to write under the tutelage of her first husband, 'Willy', under whose name the Claudine novels were originally published. In 1906 she embarked on a second career on the music hall stage, where she became associated with the Paris *demi-monde* of Natalie Clifford Barney and Renée Vivien. In 1911 she was writing for *Le Matin* and was to continue writing throughout her long life. Autobiographical themes – her mother, animals, Provence, backstage life, Paris, and learning to live with 'the beloved enemy' – reverberate throughout her novels and her occasional prose.

Her works include *Gigi, Chéri, The Vagabond, The Pure and the Impure, My Mother's House, Duo and Le Toutounier, Break of Day*, and *The Evening Star*.

**Lucy Goodison** started work at the BBC and left to become active in community-based politics. She trained in massage, and for fifteen years ran workshops in bodywork, dance and dreams at the Women's Therapy Centre in London. She is the author of *The Dreams of Women:*

*Exploring and Interpreting Women's Dreams* (The Women's Press, 1995), and co-authored (with Sheila Ernst) the bestselling *In Our Own Hands: A Book of Self-Help Therapy* (The Women's Press, 1981). She gained her doctorate for research into female religious symbolism in ancient Crete, as described in her major work *Moving Heaven and Earth: Sexuality, Spirituality and Social Change* (The Women's Press, 1990; abridged, Pandora, 1992). As a freelance journalist she specialises in issues of mental health and learning difficulties.

**Zora Neale Hurston** (1903–1960) was born in Eatonville, Florida. She won a scholarship to Barnard College, where she began her career as a folklorist. *Mules and Men* (1935) and *Tell My Horse* (1938) bring together the black traditions of the American South and the Caribbean. She also published two novels, *Their Eyes Were Watching God* (1937), and *Moses: Man of the Mountain* (1939); and an autobiography, *Dust Tracks on a Road* (1942). A collection of her writings, edited by Alice Walker, *I Love Myself When I Am Laughing* was published in 1979, and a volume of short stories, *Spank*, appeared in 1984.

**Sheila Jeffreys** is the author of *The Lesbian Heresy: A Feminist Perspective on the Lesbian Sexual Revolution* (The Women's Press, 1993); *Anticlimax: A Feminist Perspective on the Sexual Revolution* (The Women's Press, 1990); and *The Spinster and Her Enemies: Feminism and Sexuality 1880–1930* (1985). Sheila Jeffreys was a founding member of London Women Against Violence Against Women (WAVAW); and of the London Lesbian Archive, and the London Lesbian History Group. She contributed to *Not a Passing Phase: Reclaiming Lesbians in History 1840–1985* edited by the Lesbian History Group (The Women's Press, 1989), and *All the Rage: Reasserting Radical Lesbian Feminism* edited by Lynne Harne and Elaine Miller (The Women's Press, 1996); and edited *The Sexuality Debates* (1987). She is currently a Senior Lecturer in the Department of Political Science at the University of Melbourne, Australia.

**Dianne Linden** is a teacher, writer and fibre artist based in Edmonton, Alberta, Canada. Her poetry, essays and short stories have been published in a number of Canadian literary magazines, as well as on CBC Radio. 'In The Bleak Midwinter' is anthologised in *Eating Apples – Knowing Women's Lives*, and will also be buried in a timecapsule during Edmonton's Fringe Theatre Festival, to be opened in the mid-2000s. (Hopefully not bleak as well.) Currently Dianne Linden is experimenting with historical and whimsical text presented together in the context of stitchery.

**Nadezhda Mandelstam** (1899–1980) wrote two memoirs of her life with her husband Osip Mandelstam, the Russian poet sent to a Siberian concentration camp by the Communist authorities, from where his death was reported in 1938. *Hope Against Hope* was published in the West in 1970, but not until 1988 in the USSR. *Hope Abandoned* was published in 1972 in Russian in Paris, and in the United States in the same year.

**Rosemary Manning** worked in business and in teaching, and was a writer for most of her adult life.

Her novels include *Look, Stranger* (1960), *The Chinese Garden* (1962, republished 1984). *A Time and a Time*, her autobiographical account of a lesbian love affair that ended in her attempted suicide, was published under the pseudonym Sarah Davys in 1971, and reissued in 1986 under her own name. A second volume of autobiography, *A Corridor of Mirrors*, is published by The Women's Press (1987).

Among her books for children are *Green Smoke* (1957), *Dragon in Danger* (1959), *The Dragon's Quest* (1961), *Dragon in the Harbour* (1980) and *Arripay* (1963).

Rosemary Manning died in 1988.

**Marie** is a Black lesbian mother and grandmother. She was born in Barbados in 1939 but has lived most of her life in England. She is independent, has a demanding job and enjoys a happy and committed relationship with her lover, Ruth. Her main interests are in Black and feminist issues and she is keen to meet other older Black lesbians to share experiences and to socialise.

**Carol Mara** is an Australian writer. Her first book, *Eva's Crossing*, was published in 1993.

**Roberta Morris** is the author of the novels *No Words for Love and Famine* (1993), *Miriam; An Autobiography* (1993), and *Vigil* (1986). She has a masters degree in theology and is presently completing an MA in philosophy. She splits her time between New York and Toronto where she lives with her wise and beautiful daughter, Andrea, her handsome and brilliant son, Nathaniel, and his reptiles.

**Clara Piriz** had to leave her country, Uruguay, during the military regime of the 1970s. She lived in exile in Holland until the return of democracy to her country. Back in Uruguay she worked in women's organisations and graduated from university.

**Katha Pollitt**'s writing appears regularly in *The Nation, The New Yorker* and *The New Republic*. Her book of poems, *Antarctic Travellers*, won the

National Book Critics Circle Award. Her most recent work is *Reasonable Creatures*, a collection of essays. She lives in New York City.

**Sal and Anne** Sal's life has changed radically since 'Stepping Out' was written and she now lives with her male partner and one-year-old daughter. Anne says, 'Things are changing now for me for the better – I feel I'm older, wiser and better-looking!'

**Liv Ullmann** was born in 1939. She studied drama in London and began her career with a repertory company in Stavanger. She became internationally recognised as a screen actress for her roles in the films of Ingmar Bergman, including *Persona* (1966), *Cries and Whispers* (1972), *Face to Face* (1975) and *Autumn Sonata* (1978), and made her Broadway début in *A Doll's House* (1975). Her book *Changing* is translated into more than 24 languages, and a second autobiographical work, *Choices*, was published in 1984. She was appointed UNICEF Goodwill Ambassador in 1980, and has been awarded 13 honorary degrees in the Arts and Humanities, and numerous awards worldwide for her humanitarian work. She has directed the films *Kristen Lavransdatter*, and Ingmar Bergman's *Private Confessions*.

**Alice Walker** was born in Eatonton, Georgia. She has received many awards, including The Radcliffe Fellowship and a Guggenheim Fellowship. Her hugely popular novel, *The Color Purple* (The Women's Press, 1983), won the American Book Award, plus the Pulitzer Prize for Fiction in 1983, and was subsequently made into an internationally successful film by Steven Spielberg.

Alice Walker's other novels are *Meridian* (The Women's Press, 1982), of which CLR James said 'I have not read a novel superior to this'; *The Third Life of Grange Copeland* (The Women's Press, 1985); *The Temple of My Familiar* (The Women's Press, 1989), which appeared in the *New York Times* bestseller list for four months; and *Possessing the Secret of Joy* (1992). She has written two collections of short stories: *In Love and Trouble* (The Women's Press, 1984), and *You Can't Keep a Good Woman Down* (The Women's Press, 1982); and two books of essays and memoirs: *In Search of Our Mother's Gardens: Womanist Prose* (The Women's Press, 1984), and *Living by the Word* (The Women's Press, 1988). Alice Walker has published four books of poetry, all of which have been published by The Women's Press: *Horses Make a Landscape Look More Beautiful* (1985), *Once* (1986), *Good Night, Willie Lee, I'll See You in the Morning* (1987) and *Revolutionary Petunias* (1988).

Alice Walker's complete poetry is now collected together in *Her Blue Body Everything We Know: Earthling Poems 1965–1990 Complete* (1991) and her complete short stories appear in *The Complete Stories* (1994), both published by The Women's Press.

**Rebecca Walker** was born in Jackson, Mississippi, and grew up in San Francisco and New York City. She is a co-founder of the Third Wave Direct Action Corporation, a non-profit organisation dedicated to cultivating young women's leadership and activism. Her writing has appeared in *Listen Up: Voices from the Next Feminist Generation* (1995), as well as magazines such as *The Black Scholar* and *Ms.* Her first book, *To Be Real*, was published in 1995.